Take A Camel To Lunch

And Other Adventures For Mature Travelers

by Nancy O'Connell
Craig Davis, Illustrator

BRISTOL PUBLISHING ENTERPRISES, INC.
San Leandro, California

Printed in the United States of America.

ISBN 1-55867-024-6

Cover design by Frank Paredes

CONTENTS

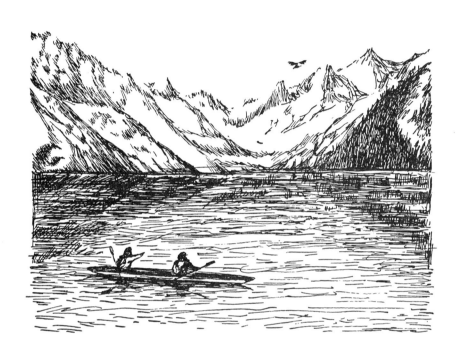

KAYAKING IN GLACIER BAY: THE FIRST OF MANY UNUSUAL ADVENTURES

We fell asleep to the thunderous sound of a gigantic glacier calving and awoke to the same primeval roar in the early morning hours. The sky had only been truly dark for about four hours, from about 11

P. M. until 3 A.M. In those few hours of darkness, certain creatures would come in close to our tents, shy creatures who did not want to be seen by man.

Our foodstuffs were stashed up on high rocks some distance from our tents. We had no wish to share our meal with a bear, nor did we wish for a nocturnal visit from this wild animal who might develop a craving for a midnight snack.

Awakening to the aroma of brewing coffee the next morning, we climbed out of our tents and spotted two killer whales a few yards away. As they emerged from the water, their black bodies glistened in the early sunlight. One was much larger than the other.

"A mother and her offspring," our guide explained, "feasting on krill."

As the great beasts again appeared on the surface of the water, we were able to make out the stark whiteness under their lower jaws and on their underbellies. They were now less than 50 feet from our campsite.

"Because they attack other mammals, the Eskimos call those whales 'sea wolves.' They hunt in packs just as the wolves do," Dave, our naturalist guide, explained.

Tracks around our bright blue tents suggested that the ptarmigan, that shy grouselike bird, had visited us in the early hours before 5 A.M. After the killer whales left the area, seals reappeared, no longer afraid, and cavorted in the water very near to us. Ice floes drifted by, some as high as three or four feet, in strange and almost mystical shapes.

The current had changed in the night. As the noisy calving continued, huge sections of shimmering blue ice fell into the bay. Overnight our route in had vanished.

"We'll have to carry our kayaks out in a different direction," our guide declared. "The path we took yesterday is blocked by ice." Near the water's edge, as we climbed closer, we watched in awe as enormous boulders of ice tumbled out into the surging waters. Some of those chunks of ice were as big as a full grown elephant seal.

Another day of adventure had commenced. Another day of pitting our puny muscles against the might of nature, another round of small personal truimphs awaited us.

Within an hour of that first sip of coffee and that first bite of pancakes, we had carried our light German-made kayaks over our heads, trudged along past rocks and over ice fields, and launched our two-man kayaks into the chilly waters of Glacier Bay, Alaska, site of one of the most spectacular of our national parks.

As I took up my paddle for the day's kayaking, I glanced at my husband and at our other companions. None of us were truly young. Only our guide was in his 30s. Two of the men had graying hair, and we women were in our 40s and 50s.

Why were we doing this? Was it for the exhilaration we felt each day as we explored a new pristine area of this icy wonderland? Was it the pride we felt at leaving no ugliness behind when we broke up camp — no record of our brief human stay there at all?

I know that each day I felt stronger, more able to keep up the pace of several hours of kayaking and exploration. Muscles which a few days before had protested were now cooperating. The natural beauty, the harmony of the sea and the glaciers — all of this comprised an experience, and later, a memory of a new achievement which has never left me.

Nine days of kayaking in Glacier Bay transformed my life. I was enriched and I was strengthened in my resolve to avoid the humdrum, to explore the world now that my children were grown, to reach out for new horizons. . .

Begin Your Own Explorations!

I have continued to reach out for new horizons and new travel adventures since those few magical days of kayaking. If you have reached that time in your life when you have an "empty nest," when the last of your children has moved out of your home, or when you have retired or for some reason have been given the gift of time, it may be the opportunity for you to begin your own unique explorations of the world.

It is now easier to travel to faraway exotic destinations than ever before. In a matter of hours you may transport yourself to any part of the world. You don't have to "rough it" in sleeping bags and tents to experience the unusual in vacation travel. Nor do you have to spend a fortune. If your resources are limited, you can still afford a vacation to Mexico where our dollar equals hundreds of pesos and where you will be immediately emersed in a culture very different from our own. Some seasoned travelers, who have made several trips to Europe, say that Mexico seems more foreign to them than England or many of the other European countries, perhaps because so many Americans are of European descent.

Another dollar stretcher could be an exchange program. You may have a desire to visit one country and study it in depth. If you are an educator, for example, you might arrange a sabbatical and teach for a year abroad. A colleague of mine who teaches at Chabot College is this year teaching in Scotland, while a Scottish professor is teaching at Chabot.

If you are seeking a shorter time abroad, and still are reeling from those college expenses for your offspring, you could arrange to exchange your home with someone in another country. The time can range from two weeks to a year. Organizations exist to match you with someone who wishes to explore your own area. You are permitted to lock up one room and label it "off limits." Hide your antiques in there and off you go! For not much more than the price of air fare, you can have an unusual adventure in a culture very different from your own.

Travel With Me

In this book I will take you around the world to various fascinating destinations. It will not be the world of luxurious cruise ships where each week 1,000 passengers visit the same port and tour the same "duty free" shop.

Nor will it be the world of $400-a-night luxury hotels where one is reminded of America, and all of the dishes served to those getting off the tour buses are identical.

Instead this will be a guide for those of you who have reached your mature years, yet are young in spirit, for those of you who wish to have unusual and offbeat adventures, for those of you who seek to travel in safety, but wish to listen to the beat of a "different drummer."

Most of these adventures do not demand great strength, nor do they test your endurance. Instead, they will appeal to anyone with a lively curiosity about peoples and places very different from his own. I have visited many of these destinations myself and later have returned with a group.

It is my sincere hope that these adventures will give you the courage to travel, to seek the unusual, and to attain through careful planning, a full and enriching exploration uniquely your own.

Explanations of Cost and Fitness Ratings

Cost ratings. Each adventure in this book will

conclude with an approximation of cost (based on the total cost of lodgings (if applicable) and activity. Since there is great variation in pricing caused by currency fluctuations and sudden changes in the world situation, the prices are meant to serve only as a guideline. You must check with your travel agent or the source I have given you at the conclusion of the adventure's description to discover the current costs.

> *inexpensive:* under $100 a day
> *moderate:* between $100 and $150 a day
> *expensive:* more than $150 a day

Fitness ratings. These ratings are designed to guide you in making a decision so that those of you who enjoy a strenuous hiking experience will not wind up on an adventure designed for those who only wish to gaze at nature through the window of a van or bus.

> *easy*: for those who enjoy strolling and are
> able to walk the length of a long city block
> *moderate*: for those who enjoy a good brisk
> walk, a minimum of climbing
> *strenuous*: for those in top physical
> condition. May require climbing or a
> tolerance for higher altitude (as stated in
> each section where applicable).

Wheelchair access. If I have read of, or observed myself, good wheelchair access, I will mention it. This information is not always available, but it is hoped that more and more companies and tour leaders will become responsive to this population.

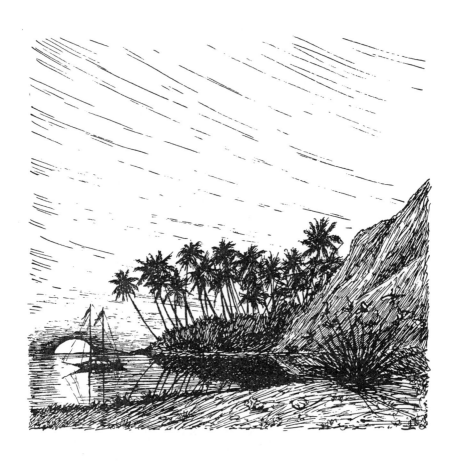

HAWAIIAN ADVENTURES

Watch a sunrise over Poipu Beach on Kauai and you will believe you have suddenly been transported into a magic world. Listen to the waves crash against the cliffs, watch the luminous colors of the clouds, and hear the barred dove and water birds call out — it will chase away all thoughts and worries of your usual life.

While on Kauai, as you erase your worries, you

will feel refreshed. But after a day spent relaxing, you will want to immerse yourself in activities quite unlike any you find back home. You will want to experience Kauai, not just lie on its beaches and become a beach bum. You have not traveled thousands of miles to vegetate. What kind of activity will you find on Hawaii's "Garden Isle?"

POIPU BEACH PARK

There are adventures to be had without exchanging any money. At Poipu Beach Park, unpack the snorkeling equipment you brought in your suitcase, and wade in a bit. Begin floating on the surface, and you will see dozens of tropical fish. In one hour our first morning of snorkeling we spotted silver aholeholes, speckled boxfish, at least three brightly colored types of parrotfish, a red-shouldered tang, wrasses, triggerfish, unicorn surgeons whose faces look like pouting old gentlemen with strange horns protruding in front of their eyes, and hundreds of trumpetfish swimming near the surface.

The next morning in the same area I had more adventure than I had envisioned. While out snorkeling I found myself staring at what looked like a big fat 26-inch long snake. It was down in the crevice of a rock under water, but as it slithered out, I took off! I had no desire to play tag with that creature, which looked big and mean and hungry. It had a dark brown body with many yellow stripes. Consulting our book on marine life forms in Hawaii, I later deduced that I had been startled by a moray eel —

the zebra moray. It did have all the stripes I have seen on zebras in Africa, but on the zebra, those stripes somehow appear friendlier.

Because of the weight, we never fly with heavy fins — goggles and a snorkel are ample for this pleasure. However, because there are some rocks here, you might want to wear a pair of those new canvas reef shoes with the rubber soles whose colors in shocking pinks and chartreuse rival the brilliance of the tropical fish.

EXPLORING KOKEE STATE PARK

Visit Kokee State Park for another free adventure. The drive is a beautiful one. Towering bougainvillea vines in muted oranges, pinks and fuchsia grow along the road as you near Hanapepe Canyon. As you start the climb, you begin to glimpse the spectacular Waimea Canyon. Waimea means *red water* and the Waimea River far below in the depths of the canyon is reddened by the iron-rich soil surrounding it.

This is not a private adventure at the main lookout point. Five tour buses laden with excited Japanese tourists arrived shortly after we did. But drive on in your rental car and you will discover other vistas where no one is parked. Take the walk off the main road, and you will encounter very few individuals.

As you approach Kokee State Park, at the fork in the road, park your car and take the Canyon Trail hike about a mile downhill. It is a gradual descent. You will be rewarded with awesome views, towering Waipoo Waterfall, and Kokee Stream where you can swim. Take a picnic; then follow the stream awhile to find the best swimming areas. You will probably be the only ones there, so take a "buddy" along. As you climb back up, stop often and enjoy the tiny wild flowers, the orange lantana, and the vistas en route. Round trip, this hike is 1.7 miles and it is rated strenuous. The altitude here is at 3,500 feet. Climbing back up the Canyon Trail one is aware of this!

After this exertion, you've earned a break. Drive on up to Kokee State Park Museum and Lodge. Enjoy a refreshing pineapple-coconut drink, and watch the dozens of native jungle fowl strutting about. Probably introduced by the Polynesians centuries ago, in late August these birds are in all their stages from newly hatched to the brilliant plummaged adult. Here also is the robin-egg blue barred dove. Visit the natural history museum with its charts and its diorama of native birds. In the late afternoon after 3 P.M., you might be the only visitors.

Note: This park is free and open to the public year around. For a full meal at the Kokee Lodge, food is served from 8:30 A.M. to 3:30 P.M. daily and dinners only on Fridays and Saturdays from 6 to 9 P.M. Kokee Lodge has a dozen small housekeeping cabins — very rustic, but fully furnished with bedding and basic cooking utensils.

Write or call:
    Kokee Lodge
    P.O. Box 819
    Waimea, Kauai, HI 96796
    (808) 335-6061
Cost: cabins are inexpensive, but must be reserved far in advance
Fitness rating: strenuous for the hiking because of the altitude, but minimal around the Kokee State Park Museum
Wheelchair access: a ramp leads to the lodge and to main lookout point

HELICOPTER "FLIGHT-SEEING" OVER KAUAI

To truly see some of the inaccessible areas of Kauai, a unique and memorable way to visit the rugged terrain is to fly over it. You could be in that tiny helicopter you spied down in Waimea Canyon while you were viewing the canyon along with five busloads of Japanese tourists!

That tiny helicopter appears much bigger up close and transports you to some breathtaking views of not only the famous canyon, but the cliffs of Na Pali, and the center of Mt. Waialeae's crater. Kauai is the oldest of Hawaii's islands, but it too had its beginnings from a volcano's eruption — Mt. Waialeale — Kauai's long extinct volcano.

You will be close enough to see mountain goats, the snowy egrets which hover in flocks over the sugar cane, and numerous waterfalls close to their sources.

There is no location in the world boasting of more

rain than Mt. Waialeae, so check the weather reports before making your reservation. Flights will be rescheduled if there is inclement weather or poor visibility, and your money will be refunded if you are leaving the next day.

You might also want to check ahead with the Federal Aviation Administration in Honolulu. Ask which companies have air-taxi certificates; ask for their safety records. There are now many helicopter companies operating in Kauai and you will want to choose the most reliable.

Write or call:
　　　Papillon Hawaiian Helicopters
　　　P.O. Box 339
　　　Hanalei, HI 96714
　　　(808) 245-9644

Cost: inexpensive to moderate. Prices vary according to length of time in the air. Some companies offer a champagne luncheon near a mountain stream. This would naturally be more costly.

Fitness rating: easy

Wheelchair access: probably not, but your "significant other" could help you into the craft

BIRDING ON KAUAI:
VISIT KILAUEA POINT WILDLIFE REFUGE

In 1909, Teddy Roosevelt was farsighted enough to establish the Hawaiian Island National Wildlife Refuge. Today it includes some 1,800 acres of land and tiny atolls spread over many miles between Nihoa Island and Pearl and Hermes Reef in northwest Hawaii. Some are only tiny dots in the enormous Pacific Ocean, but taken collectively, are home to more than fourteen million seabirds! Kilauea Point National Wildlife Refuge is a small portion of this vast Hawaiian Island National Wildlife Refuge. At Kilauea Point National Wildlife Refuge, if you are an avid birder you will enjoy seeing the great frigatebirds soaring above you. With a zoom or a telephoto lens you could get some excellent photos. The frigatebirds are called thieves or *iwa* by the Hawaiians. They frighten the red-footed boobies and shearwaters here and steal their food. (In the Galapagos Islands I saw evidence of them stealing tortoise eggs.)

Thousands of red-footed boobies were nesting here in August, but only a strong telephoto lens would give you a good look. Or, arrive early and go on a two-mile docent-led hike. There are several scheduled each day. Then, you will get much closer to the nesting areas of the laysan albatross, the boobies, or the wedge-tailed shearwaters as you hike along the Crater Hill coastline. One public tour you can count on is daily at noon, except on Saturdays.

From January through March, you may see humpback whales swimming and breaching nearby.

Of interest is the Kiluea Lighthouse, built in 1913, now on the National Register of Historic Places.

To get to the Kilauea Point National Wildlife Refuge, drive one mile from Kilauea, following a good map. Just when you are certain you are lost, you will come upon it. Hours are 10:00 A.M. to 4 P. M.

Write or call:
Kilauea Point National Wildlife Refuge
P.O. Box 87,
Kilauea, Kauai, HI 96754
(808) 828-1525
Cost: $2.00 per family — a bargain
Fitness rating: easy
Wheelchair access: possible. A wheelchair could be pushed up the gentle slope; then there are long level stretches of good pavement. With binoculars, this refuge could bring nature up close to the viewer.

CAPTAIN ZODIAC RAFTING ADVENTURES

During the winter months, Captain Zodiac operates rafts to whale watch off Kauai near the wild and uninhabited Na Pali Coast region. There are no roads here. Only a few courageous hikers can traverse this area. Because of the location and the high amount of rainfall, the paths are often muddy and very slippery.

But if you sign up for a four-hour exploration of the Na Pali area with Captain Zodiac, you will probably see giant sea turtles, a dolphin or two, and in certain winter months, humpback whales.

His motorized raft can maneuver in and out of caves. You'll see where one of the James Bond movies was filmed. You'll stop breathing as the raft rushes into a darkened cave and then slows down in the quiet blackness of the cave's depths. The official reason for this acceleration is that the captain can more easily control the craft when buzzing along at top speed.

This trip is suitable for all ages, as long as the passengers can swim. I was with several people in their late 70s and their delight in this adventure was just as keen as for those a fraction of their age. The last half hour of the Zodiac tour in Kauai is spent snorkeling at a nearly deserted beach which is remote and spectacularly beautiful. The equipment for snorkeling is provided.

The Zodiac is a craft developed originally for Jacques Cousteau and is virtually unsinkable. It can hold from ten to fourteen passengers.

Write or call:
> Captain Zodiac Rafting Expeditions
> P.O. Box 456
> Hanalei, Kauai 96714
> (808) 826-9371

Cost: inexpensive

Fitness rating: easy, but the ability to swim will make the adventure more enjoyable

CAPTAIN ZODIAC
ON THE BIG ISLAND OF HAWAII

Captain Zodiac also operates a rafting expedition on the Kona Coast on the big island, Hawaii. The adventure on this island departs from Honokohau Harbor and passengers are picked up on the piers of Kailua and Keauhou. Again the excursion lasts about four hours. You view the Kona Coastline, sea caves and grottos. After you come to the monument erected in Captain Cook's memory, you swim and snorkel. The snorkeling equipment is provided and this tour includes a tropical lunch.

Whale watching during the season of the year when the humpback whale is migrating is also offered. Generally this migration begins in January and lasts through the first half of March. Sometimes the time varies by two or three weeks, and the whales can be seen in the Lahaina area of Maui from November until May in some years.

Write or call:
Captain Zodiac Rafting Expeditions
P.O. Box 5612
Kailua-Kona, HI 96740
(800) 247-1484
Cost: inexpensive
Fitness rating: easy

More About Whale Watching

Just as the Alaskan workers and shop owners, who work all summer in Alaska, vacation in Hawaii during the winter, the humpback whales migrate to Lahaina, Maui, and other parts of Hawaii after spending their summers voraciously eating in the Bering Sea.

The whales, like some humans, seem to like siestas. At any rate, whether they are sleeping or just submerged, they are most visible to humans between 8 A.M. and 11 A.M. and from 1:30 P.M. to 5 P.M.

North of Wailea and Kihei and south of Lahaina is Maalaea Bay. Here humpback whales come in the winter and early spring months to breed. They have found their way to the island of Maui all the way from the Arctic waters of Alaska. While here in Hawaiian waters, their usual pattern is to swim from Maalaea to above Lahaina, then west to Molokai and Lanai. Only then do they swim back to Maalaea Bay.

In Lahaina, Maui, these endangered creatures are studied by several organizations. You may call Whale Report Center (808) 661-8527 for the daily sightings.

Sea Bird Cruises (808) 661-3643 and Windjammer Cruises (808) 667-6834, both operate whale viewing cruises out of Lahaina.

Other companies which offer whale watching excursions are Ocean Sports at Waikoloa on the Big Island, which combines whale watching with its snorkeling and sunset tours, and The Pacific Whale Foundation, (808) 924-5311, which also operates whale watching tours daily during this season. These tours depart from Kailua Bay.

CAPTAIN BEAN'S CRUISES

I first explored Kealakekua Bay near Captain Cook's Monument with one of Captain Bean's cruises, and the amount and variety of tropical fish in this bay near the monument rival the variety I've seen in the Great Barrier Reef in Australia.

Captain Bean's Kealakekua Bay Snorkel Cruise has a bigger boat and offers glass bottom viewing so that landlubbers can enjoy the feeding frenzy when a diver drops into the cool waters and feeds the waiting horde.

waiting horde.

When you view the three unfurled red sails of Captain Bean's *Tamure* and the impressive hull, you know you are in for an adventure. The catamaran is designed to be like the double hulled canoes which the ancient Polynesians used. When you look at her decks you will see tapa patterns based on early petroglyphs.

A light lunch is optional, as are beer, soft drinks, and snacks. Snorkeling gear is provided.

The crew aboard is particularly helpful. They go into the water with the snorkelers, and I remember their patience in teaching Mother, a good strong swimmer, but a young 80-year-old novice to snorkeling, the joy of this sport.

Write or call:
> Captain Bean's Cruises
> 74-5626 Alapa St., Bldg. B, #17
> Kailua-Kona, HI 96745
> (808) 329-2955

Cost: inexpensive; half price for children 12 years and under

Fitness rating: moderate; ability to swim will increase your pleasure

A Tip About Snorkeling Gear

As I may have explained earlier, I prefer to carry my own mask and breathing tube, or snorkel. Over and over again, I used to be given the wrong fit with the mask. Ten miles out to sea, and $15 poorer, my mask would constantly fill with salty water, my eyes would sting, and my vision would be obscured. If good snug fit. Even though many companies like Captain Bean provide you with snorkeling equipment at no extra cost beyond their initial charge, they might not have your size.

Or, for $15 per week, rent the equipment from Snorkel Bob's, located on each major Hawaiian island. This company even has prescription goggles!

SCUBAIR

A new type of sport I've never personally tried is called Scubair. It blends some of the thrills of diving with a mask and a breathing hose which runs up to oxygen supplies on the ship. It is advertised as easier to learn than snorkeling, because you don't have to master a breathing technique. You can dive deeper than when snorkeling and with the aid of flippers, you can probably range quite far from the boat. A certified, or NAUI (National Association of Underwater Instructors) instructor is on board to help you. Near the Kona coast, the company will arrange to pick you up at your hotel.

Call:
Scubair
(808) 322-6665
Cost: inexpensive
Fitness rating: moderate

SNORKELING IN THE KONA AREA

We were delighted to discover excellent snorkeling on our first morning in the Kona area of the big island of Hawaii. People travel from all over the world to visit Kona for snorkeling and diving; but I did not expect to see such an infinite variety at a beach which was so accessible.

Mothers bring their babies and toddlers, honeymooners laze on the beach, and seasoned, hardy adventurers in their retirement years line the beach and venture in with their snorkeling gear or with equipment rented out on the premises. Kahaluu Beach Park, just a few miles south of Kailua, is excellent for all ages and all levels of swimmers.

The mothers would wade in, holding their toddlers, who clutched a bag of frozen peas. Babies, also in their mother's arms, would squeal with delight, as would the toddlers, as myriad fish approached and began to gulp down the peas.

One toddler was even teaching her small black puppy to use a boogie board!

But beyond the toddlers and the honeymooners, the serious snorkeler can float face downward for a half hour to an hour at a time, without having to surface once. It is a magical quiet out there, with only the fish and your swimming buddy.

Some of the fish we saw out in this semi-private realm of water were the same as we saw in the Poipu Beach area of Kauai, but we saw others as well. The yellow and black long-nosed butterflyfish with his very long snout, the colorful lined butterflyfish, and three or four other butterflyfish, including the brilliant citron-yellow lemon butterflyfish and the raccoon butterflyfish, named because its face resembles a raccoon.

The goatfishes were numerous. The weke was easy to spot because of its whiskers, and as it fed off the bottom of the sea, a flurry of sand would scatter in all directions. The moorish idol, the various parrotfishes, the fat tiny pufferfish which looked blown up like a balloon, the many tangs and triggerfish, all made us want to go back again and again.

When a school of big 24-inch scribbled filefish swam towards us, showing all of their teeth, however, we swam away. They probably were only expecting a free dinner of frozen peas from us, but we had nothing for them, and they looked hungry and too much like panhandlers expecting a free handout.

More About Snorkeling

Here are some safety precautions to exercise while snorkeling anywhere in the world:

- Swim with a "buddy." You don't have to cling to one another, but remain within 10 or 20 feet — close enough to detect a problem if one of you is having difficulties and needs help.
- When in doubt about whether a fish is "friendly" or not, swim away and find a new space. Remember, fish are territorial.
- Never turn your back on the sea.
- Put on a good sunblock. Skin cancer is more common now than it used to be. Slather the sunblock all over your exposed areas and

especially on your face, your back and the back of your thighs and lower legs.

Snorkeling is far better for you than sunbathing. Your face, the most susceptible part of your body to develop skin cancer, is submerged in the water while snorkeling and thus is protected from the sun's rays. Don't just stand knee deep in the water for a half hour as I do, like a "Casper Milktoast," exposing yourself to the sun's rays. Jump in and immediately enjoy the wonders of the undersea world.

If you are snorkeling in Can Cun, Hawaii, or Acapulco, remember you are closer to the equator and will sunburn more readily than at home. If you are fair-skinned or a redhead, exercise caution. Snorkel early in the morning and after 3:30 P.M.

A HELICOPTER RIDE OVER THE WORLD'S MOST ACTIVE VOLCANO

If your time is limited on the big island of Hawaii, and you want to view Kilauea, the live volcano that is still destroying houses and spewing forth glowing red hot lava, you would enjoy a helicopter tour over this cauldron of molten lava.

The viewer is not only awestruck by the forces unleashed by Kilauea's fiery eruptions, he is also made aware that this island is the newest land on earth and it is still changing, still evolving with each new flow of molten lava. The magnificent Black Sands

Beach, once one of the most photographed beaches in the world, has almost totally vanished.

Yet new black sand beaches are forming as the hot lava races into the cold waters of the sea. This cold water splinters and shatters the lava into tiny black particles of sand.

The ancient Polynesians worshipped the volcano. Pele, the goddess of fire, was a deity greatly to be feared, yet she was also revered. It was their belief that Pele was an ancestor who lived on as a guardian spirit. When she became angry, her fury was unleased in a volcanic eruption.

Between 1983 and 1986 alone, more than 48 eruptive phases have originated from Kilauea, and it is still spouting forth fire.

Take a good camera on this helicopter tour, one that will photograph the detail you will want to preserve in your memory.

From Hilo at least three firms offer these flights:

- 'Io Aviation calls their flight "Helicopter Photo Flights" and has video cameras for rent. Call (808) 935-3031.
- Kaino Aviation offers a one-hour helicopter tour of the volcano. Call (808) 961-5591.
- Papillon offers 80-90 minute aerial tours of the geysers of fire from the volcano. Call (800) 367-7095.

A STAY IN VOLCANO HOUSE
If you have time and do not care to ride in a

helicopter, I would recommend a night or two spent at Volcano House, which is located in the very large Volcanoes National Park. When I first visited this hotel, I was reminded of the Ahwahnee at Yosemite National Park. From the dining room or the cocktail lounge you may see an eruption of fire shooting up from Kilauea's crater. This fiery display will eclipse all man-made fireworks you have ever seen. Volcano House has a fireplace built of lava rock, and guests gather around this area to talk and to read. Since the 1870s, when the first Volcano House was built, it has been a tradition that the fire in this fireplace never is allowed to die out.

Bundle up, because your evenings are cold at this 4,000-foot elevation, but this fire will help to keep you warm. Or, if you wish to elevate your body temperature quickly, this hotel offers a sauna heated by the steam vents from the volcano! That sounds like it would warm up the devil himself.

Write or call:
  Volcano House Hotel
  P.O. Box 53
  Hawaii Volcanoes National Park, HI 96718
  (808) 967-7321
Cost: inexpensive. If you wish to continue gazing at the volcano, ask for a superior or a deluxe room at approximately $50.00 more per night per room. Standard rooms are located behind the main hotel and do not have a view of the volcano.
Fitness rating: easy
Wheelchair access: probably

PRIVATE YACHT CHARTERS ON KONA

Are you a good sailor? One who doesn't get seasick just thinking of the open sea? Then you might enjoy chartering a private yacht for a week. (If one of the members of your family does fight seasickness, but the rest of you enjoy it immensely, talk to your family doctor. Those "Transderm Scops" containing scopolamine come in the form of tiny disks. Placed behind the ear, they will keep one shipshape for three full days, but are available only by prescription.)

Kona Aggressor, with departures from the Kailua-Kona Pier, offers many features aboard the private yachts it charters on a weekly basis: unlimited diving, a photo lab on board, a sundeck, a hot tub, and a galley with a professional chef. Your cabins have private bath and shower.

Call:

    Kona Aggressor
    (808) 344-KONA

Cost: moderate — no more than most cruises which you share with perhaps 1,500 people!

MULE RIDE ON MOLOKAI

At one time the island of Molokai in Hawaii was associated with the dreaded disease of leprosy. Now the illness is called Hansen's disease, can be arrested with drugs, and is known to be much less contagious than was believed over a hundred years ago when sufferers of this disease were dumped near the island of Molokai in Waikolu Bay. They either sank while at sea and perished, or swam ashore and somehow survived, living out their unhappy lives in the area known as the Kalaupapa Peninsula.

Today the Kalaupapa Peninsula is still an isolated area on the northern part of Molokai, but it has been made into a National Historical Park. It is now peaceful and serene, an escape from the 20th century's world of rushing, overcrowding and traffic jams.

Tourists like to explore this secluded park by riding in on the celebrated Molokai Mule Ride. The trail has at least 26 "switch-backs" through rugged terrain and underbrush that was first slashed away and cleared as a path by the Portuguese immigrant Manuel Farinha. Since he completed his task in 1886, the trail has been improved, but it still is basically his trail that is traveled.

Rare Adventures organizes these day-long expeditions, but the excitement is not limited to just the mule ride. One does not spend eight hours atop a mule!

The day begins at 8 A.M. and the group arrives at Kalaupapa after about an hour and a half of riding. As the trail descends down 1,600 feet, the rider is treated to views of the ocean glimpsed below. Forests and wild flowers are seen as you traverse back and forth in a zigzag line downwards.

By the time you reach the sea, another guide appears and the group is transported in vans for a picnic lunch. Afterward you visit the St. Philomena Church and the group hears a talk on the work of Father Damien, the Belgian priest who lived among those who suffered from leprosy. His compassion gave the patients the will to live again.

This, then, is an adventure which provides food for both your body and your soul as you realize how great a difference this one good man made in the lives of others.

Write or call:
> Rare Adventures Ltd.
> (808)553-3311
>   or
> Molokai Mule Ride
> P.O. Box 200
> Kualapuu, Molokai, HI 96757
> (808) 567-6088

Cost: inexpensive
Fitness rating: moderate

MAUI DOWNHILL

If your idea of a splendid time is to be awakened by a jangling alarm at 3 A.M., to sleepily climb into a van at 4 A.M. as it rounds up fellow adventurers at their hotels and condos, and then to head for an exercise you may not have indulged in for more than 20 or 30 years, then this is the adventure for you.

Actually it will be exciting and you will be surrounded by natural beauty. Does that make it sound more palatable?

Friends in their early 50s have raved about this experience to me, but since I love to stay up late reading, thus far they have not persuaded me to try it. I am more prone to retiring at 1 A.M. than I am to arising at 3 A.M., particularly on Maui, that tropical paradise.

How long has it been since you rode a bicycle? No fair counting that exercycle gathering dust in a corner of your TV room, I mean a *real* bicycle.

Yes, that is going to be your conveyance on this trip. Bundle up in layers after you climb out of that warm nest at 3 A.M., for you will be climbing, in that van which picks you up at 4 A.M., from sea level to the top of the spectacular Haleakala Crater at 10,000 feet.

As you climb out of the van, you will shiver in the early morning cold and pull on another sweater, but you will be awestruck by the rugged beauty of Haleakala at sunrise. In Hawaiian the very name Haleakala evokes the sun, for it means *House of the Sun.*

The silversword, a plant found nowhere else in the world, shimmers with diffused light at this hour. The colors in the sands rival Arizona's Painted Desert.

After you mount your bicycles to descend into the bowels of the crater, check your brakes. They are guaranteed to be in excellent working order. Remember the altitude and drink liquids before setting off.

As you descend, you and your group follow your guide single file. Keep your eyes on your path as you coast downhill (advice I can give with fervor, since I once had an accident I'll never forget, admiring a canal in Germany while riding a bike). A van follows the group and is in radio contact with the guide leading the way.

As your group descends, you travel through eucalyptus forests and come to flowers and later fields of vegetables. All of you stop for a picnic lunch and then you bike on to two small towns — Makawao and Paia — where you can purchase a cool and refreshing drink.

The experience lasts seven hours. After your arrival back in your hotel, you'll probably opt for a nap, yet for months thereafter you'll be telling your friends about this invigorating and unique adventure while night owls like myself will tell you how magnificent Haleakala Crater is at sunset.

One suggestion might be to book this ahead of time with your travel agent for the day after your arrival on Maui. There is a three-hour time change from California and a six-hour one from the East Coast. A 3 A.M. alarm would not be such a shock to your system immediately after your arrival. You might groggily reach for your grey flannel suit thinking it is a working day, but when you touch your jeans instead, or your wet bathing suit, you'll know you are on vacation.

Write or call:
    Maui Downhill
    333 Dairy Road, Suite 201E
    Kahului, Maui HI 96733

(808) 871-2155
or
Cruiser Bob's
(808) 677-7717
Cost: inexpensive
Fitness rating: strenuous

HALEAKALA AFOOT OR ON HORSEBACK

Another way to explore Haleakala Crater might be on horseback. Two companies offer these guided excursions.

Call:

Rainbow Ranch Riding Stables
(808) 669-4991
or
Pony Express Tours
(808) 667-2202

For vigorous outdoors types there are also over 32 miles of hiking trails within this enormous crater.

Thus, you may explore Haleakala on your own two feet, on the four hooves of your borrowed horse, or on the two wheels of a rented bicycle. The choice is yours.

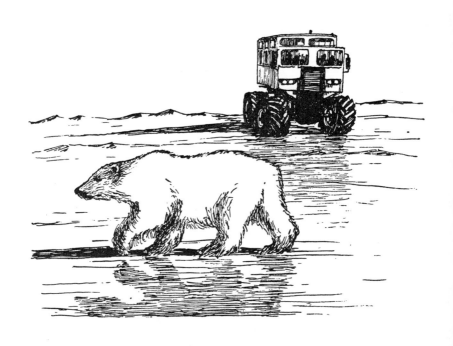

ADVENTURES
IN THE WORLD
OF ICE AND SNOW

Have you ever longed to ski in July or August, longed for that feeling of soaring effortlessly down a mountain slope covered with fresh snow? I used to have such dreams when our temperatures in California climbed to over 100°.

You can realize those dreams by visiting your favorite travel agent and booking a flight to Chile or New Zealand. You have heard that South America has warm temperatures and is often hot? True, but south of the equator the seasons are the reverse of North America's. When we're experiencing summer, it is winter for the people of Chile.

THE PORTILLO RESORT
Fly into Santiago, Chile and take a bus or a taxi from the Santiago International Airport to Portillo. This ride lasts about two and a half hours.

Portillo is a resort high up in the Andes very near the border of Argentina. The Portillo Resort overlooks a beautiful lake, Laguna del Inca. Although the resort was built about 40 years ago, it has added features which would appeal to health enthusiasts — saunas, an outdoor swimming pool, a skating rink, and a gym. The lounge has apres-ski ambience. Cocktails are served in a large room with wood paneling and a big fireplace.

Renovated in 1987, this is considered one of the best resorts in South America. There are three restaurants on the premises with international cuisine. If you want to sample typical Chilean food, the town of La Posada is a short walk from the resort.

Everything is geared to the skier here, so if you don't ski, there is not much planned activity for you. However, for the avid skier, there are some famous runs, as well as beginning and intermediate slopes. Portillo has a ski school headed by the director of the one at Heavenly Valley in California. That sounds like a very pleasant commute. He must spend the winter months in California and the summer months in Chile.

Heli-skiing (which is also popular in New Zealand) at the time of this writing was $700 in Chile for an hour's trip for five people. For this adventure, a helicopter transports you way up into the stratosphere and then you ski down.

Write or fax:

Hotel Portillo Reservation Office
Roger de Flor
2911, Santiago, Chile
FAX 56-2-231-7164

Cost: moderate to expensive. Rates at the resort are all inclusive — they include all meals, and tea for those who can't hold out for 9 P.M. dining, seven all-day lift passes, plus a half-day pass for your first day of arrival. For the budget minded, one can rent bunks in a room without a private bath. Children under 4 are free and if they are under 12 years, the rate is one-half of the adult fare when the room is shared with the parent or grandparent.

Fitness rating: moderate to strenuous

For information about skiing in our summer months in New Zealand, see page 99.

CROSS-COUNTRY SKIING

People of all ages are on the slopes. At Squaw Valley in California I have met 70-year-olds who are enthusiastic about the sport. Skiing in Innsbruch and on its many slopes, not only were many of the men gray-haired and obviously in their late 60s, but three or four of them with only one leg would schuss past me on the slopes.

Since I broke my ankle skiing when a big mountain of a man plowed into me from above and behind me, I have been cautious. I was intimidated my first time back on skis when an entire school of first, second, and third graders raced by me on their skis in Halloween costumes — witches flew past, as did giant fat pumpkins, and delightful goblins — masks and all.

Many of my friends have turned to cross-country skiing as they move up the corporate or academic ladders and realize they can no longer risk a broken limb and a month or two of discomfort. The areas I mention in this book certainly welcome the cross-country skier, as well as the downhill daredevil. In addition, several areas cater especially to the cross-country skier.

CROSS-COUNTRY SKIING IN FINLAND

If you travel to Finland in the winter months, you can participate in many unusual adventures. As in Alaska, you can mush forward on a "Husky Safari." Let the dogs transport you through the snow while you are relaxed on a sleigh driven by an expert, or you may elect to drive the sleigh yourself.

How about a ride in a sleigh pulled by a reindeer in Lapland? These are clever creatures and many are well trained to the harness. Here also, you can take over the reins and steer along trails or adventure out into the snowy wilderness where the recently fallen snow makes the land pristine. You will then feel as though you are the first human to explore this white wilderness.

If you like to fish, ice fishing is offered here. Fishing holes are drilled in the ice and the Laplanders catch perch or turbot. If you are from the northeastern part of the United States, this might remind you of your own youth and not be so appealing.

However, what does sound appealing and is a great favorite with those who reside in Finland is cross-country skiing. For a long while this has been one of their modes of winter travel. Unlike downhill skiing, which carries some risk of broken bones if one experiences a nasty fall, cross-country skiing is safe and anyone of any age can participate as long as he enjoys good health. A different type of ski, boot and binding is used from the downhill skiing equipment, and if one can walk, one can learn to cross-country ski.

The joy in this type of skiing is that a group can explore areas far from a crowd. There is no waiting in long lines at the ski lifts. The comradery that springs up in a congenial group exploring a winter wonderland of snow and ice is terrific.

Relax after a day of cross-country skiing with that Finnish institution, the sauna. At one time in Finland, a sauna was the place for a baby to be born. It must have been a warm and womblike temperature for the newborn! In today's world, it is here that one is supposed to relax. Just as most of us have been told it's not polite to argue while dining, the Finns have been told that while in the sauna there should be no display of bad temper.

After bathing in the sauna, the real men of Finland do not eat quiche, they roll in the snow or swim in one of their many cold, cold lakes. In the southern part of Finland, that area alone boasts of 30,000 lakes.

If you wish to ski in Finland, you can count on snow from the middle of October. In northern Lapland, which is a province of Finland above the Arctic Circle, you can also count on a very strange phenomenon — the *kaamos*. During December and January the sun does not appear at all. One merely sees a glimmer of its rays beyond the horizon.

Yet, despite this eerie effect, Lapland features many good cross-country skiing facilities. One can see clearly enough for that sport even during *kaamos*; and in the evening, the ski tracks are illuminated, as are the downhill slopes.

You can choose to stay in hotels or motels or travel to remote villages and stay in small detached log cabins, taking your meals in a village restaurant.

Instruction in cross-country skiing is available at almost every ski center in Finland. It is easy to rent equipment. For a multi-lingual guide and a planned itinerary where all of your belongings are moved on to the next stop, as in the walking tours in Europe, book through a travel agent. Finnair has good flights to Helsinki out of New York and good add-on fares from the West Coast.

Write or call:
> Finnair
> 10 East 40th Street
> New York, NY 10016
> (212) 689-9300

Cost: (inexpensive) for rental of cross-country skis, poles and boots — no need for a lift ticket! Airfares to Finland are considerably lower through the winter months than during the summer high season. Finland's proximity to Russia has made Finnair one of the favored carriers for travelers to that enormous neighbor in the popular summer months, but the demand is lower in the winter — a good reason for enjoying Finland as a destination of its own.

CROSS-COUNTRY SKIING
IN AMERICA AND CANADA

If you wish to conquer cross-country skiing, you may enjoy it without traveling abroad, of course. Some areas where it is a very popular sport in America: Mount Bachelor in Oregon, Crystal Mountain Resort in Washington, Jackson Hole, Wyoming, and Kirkwood, 30 miles south of Lake Tahoe, in California. Read on for a thumbnail sketch of each of those four destinations.

Mt. Bachelor

Mt. Bachelor is a volcano cone which stretches up to 9,065 feet. At its base is Deschutes National Forest. One can usually ski here until late spring.

The resort area is located 22 miles southwest of Bend, Oregon.

Call: Mt. Bachelor Ski and Summer Resort
(503) 382-8334

Crystal Mountain Resort

This resort is on Mt. Rainier at the 3,900 foot level. Downhill skiing can be from a summit at 7,000 feet, but at the various altitudes cross-country skiers will find more than 1,000 acres through the back country for their enjoyment. Located 67 miles from the Seattle Airport, it is easy to reach with a rental car equipped with snow tires.

Call: Crystal Mountain Resort, Washington
(206) 663-2265

Jackson Hole, Wyoming

Jackson Hole boasts its own airport and several carriers fly directly into this mecca for skiers. It offers more than 100 miles of runs and encompasses more than 2,500 acres. The area of Teton Village, at the base of the 10,450 foot summit, provides for ideal cross-country skiing. Trails at the base can lead those who wish to explore nature into Grand Teton National Park. For those downhill skiers with a yen for adventure, helicopter skiing is offered on three different mountain ranges near Jackson Hole.

Do you want to take an old-fashioned sleigh ride? Here is one area where this is offered. View some of the thousands of elk which winter here beneath the Grand Tetons, or put ear muffs on to deaden the sound of the motor, and take a snowmobile ride into Yellowstone National Park.

Call: Jackson Hole Ski Resort
(307) 733-2292

Kirkwood

Kirkwood is the most southern of Tahoe's ski areas. It is a three-and-a-half hour drive north from San Francisco, California. You can also fly into Lake Tahoe Airport, weather permitting, rent a car, and drive the 30 miles to Kirkwood. This resort boasts an average of 425 inches of snow a year. One can usually ski here from November until the middle of May.

Kirkwood is at 9,800 feet, so that may be too high an altitude for everyone. The Nordic sport of cross-country skiing here has 80 kilometers of well prepared trails, along with signs that tell the skier which wild animals have been seen recently in the area.

Call: Kirkwood Ski Resort
(209) 258-6000

In Canada, one can cross-country ski at Lake Louise in Alberta where there are 50 miles of cross-country trials, or at Marmot Basin, also in Alberta. At Marmot Basin there are well defined cross-country skiing tracks, ice fishing and dog sledding. (Did some Finns move here earlier in the century?)

MORE ICE AND SNOW ADVENTURES:
SEEKING POLAR BEARS

While in Canada you might like to visit the "Polar Bear Capital" of the world in Churchill, Manitoba. If you stay overnight in this small port located a full 1,000 miles north of Chicago, you might encounter a polar bear rummaging through a local garbage can. Don't panic. It might be a mother out foraging for food for her cubs nearby.

The polar bears were here first. For centuries these large white carnivores have migrated through this area and the presence of man has not deterred them. Years ago the bears were shot and killed if they came too close to humans, but now the great white beasts are captured and removed to a safe area further away from human civilization.

Just report that errant bear from the safety of your hotel lobby and the lumbering intruder will be rescued. You wouldn't want the streets to be unsafe at night, would you? That might be too much like being at home.

A company called Natural Wildlife Adventures offers a series of polar bear watching adventures slated for the fall months during the period of the great annual migration of approximately 1,500 polar bears.

Have you ever ridden in a tundra buggy or even seen one? The passengers ride up high in a strange conveyance that looks like a cross between a tank and a land rover with many big windows. This is set atop huge truck-like tires with enormous treads. You sit up as high as you would riding on an elephant.

From the safety of your tundra buggy, you view these great mammals in their natural habitat, see the baby cubs cavorting in the snow, and delight in their antics in the arctic. This "soft" adventure lasts for seven nights and originates in Winnipeg, Canada. The package includes local air flights, hotel accommodations, meals, three days of tundra buggy excursions, a guide and a professional photographer or naturalist.

Since the tundra buggy must be heated, it sounds like a great adventure! When you return home you might put yourself to sleep counting all the bears you saw, rather than sheep.

Call: Natural Habitat Wildlife Adventures
(201) 209-4747
Cost: expensive
Fitness rating: easy; the first step is a steep one, however
Wheelchair access: no

ANTARCTICA:
SOUTHERN LAND OF ICE AND SNOW

For many people, Antarctica holds a fascination, a pull that is difficult for others to fathom. Perhaps it is partially that it is considered to be the Last Continent, the one least visited by man, the last one to open up to tourists at all.

For a long while, only research scientists were allowed into Antarctica to make scientific studies. Perhaps the lure and excitement is there because it was forbidden to the rest of us for so long.

Only a few tourists are allowed in each year during the summer months in the southern hemisphere — January and February. Instead of being in darkness most of the time, it is now light for 20 hours each day.

Mountain Travel, an adventure company which has been organizing unusual walking and hiking tours for many years, offers a cruise experience aboard the *M.V. Illiria* in mid-February.

The itinerary is exciting. Everyone flies into Buenos Aires, Argentina and will meet there in this cosmopolitan city. A day will be spent exploring the city and then everyone will fly south across fields of pampas to Rio Grande. From here they will be driven to Ushuaia, a town which is further south than any other in the world.

Boarding the *M.V. Illiria*, which has now cruised the Antartic for three seasons, the travelers will settle into their cabins. There are 90 officers and stewards on board, and the capacity is for 140 guests. Boasting a library, a lounge, a card room, and a doctor's office, the vessel offers other amenities like a gym, a swimming pool, a promenade deck and a hairdresser. In April of 1990 this ship was extensively refurbished. It is the ship often chosen by universities for their study tours and alumni group cruises where learning accompanies traveling. There is *one seating* for dinner. This is highly civilized. Everyone can dine at the same time, so there is no need to gulp down your dessert and scald your tongue on your last cup of coffee because other voyagers are ravenous and want you to clear out of the dining room.

The group will hear lectures on board, as they sail through the Beagle Channel, which was described by Darwin in 1832 while aboard the *Beagle.* The ship will head towards Cape Horn, a small island discovered by a Dutch navigator in 1616, and then cover the 600 miles to Antarctica. Albatross and petrels fly overhead, and as the group gets closer to Antarctica, whales and rare penguins will be seen — penguins with brilliant tufts of feathers on their heads.

A stop will be made at Deception Island, an active volcano. The group will visit various research stations and will make other stops depending upon weather conditions.

On the minus side, there could be storms at sea, and this is a small ship. Mountain Travel asks that all of its passengers be in good physical shape for this adventure and that they enjoy roughing it.

For exploring areas too narrow for the *Illiria,* rubber Zodiacs which seat twelve people will be employed. Penguin rookeries and other wild life will come into close viewing range because of the versalitity of these Zodiacs.

Heading back, the group will disembark in Ushuaia and visit Tierra del Fuego National Park, which encompasses 155,000 acres. Members of the Audubon Society will enjoy the unusual bird life to be found here.

A flight back to Buenos Aires and then a day spent in acclimatizing oneself to civilization once more will help the travelers unwind from the natural high they will be on after such a thrilling experience. Then will come the long flight home.

However, if you wish one more adventure before leaving this area, arrangements can be made in advance with your travel agent or with Mountain Travel for you to visit Iguazu Falls, the largest waterfall in the world.

Like Society Expeditions, which also offers a tour to Antarctica, Mountain Travel is dedicated to preserving the environment. It states on its brochure: "Wildlife and habitats of the Antarctic are protected by the Antarctic Treaty, which governs all activity below 60° south. Our visits are arranged so that we do not disturb nesting seabirds or disrupt vital research."

Write or call:
> Mountain Travel
> 6420 Fairmount Ave.,
> El Cerrito, CA 94530
> (415) 527-8100

Cost: expensive
Fitness rating: moderate to strenuous
Wheelchair access: no

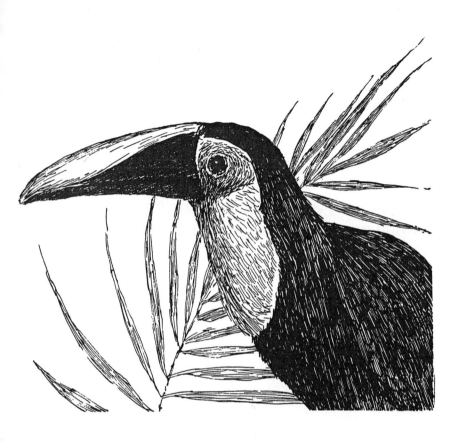

EXPLORING THE ORINOCO RIVER

If you are able to afford it and enjoy unusual destinations and natural beauty far from civilization, you would enjoy a cruise with Society Expeditions. People of all ages can travel with this company knowing that it is very reliable, has thoroughly researched the area to be explored, and is meticulous in its planning.

It has mouth watering itineraries for those who long for the extraordinary adventure. You will feel like an explorer who has ventured into areas of the world which few Americans or Europeans have been privileged to visit.

Society Expeditions does not appeal to the masses. Their ships are not for those who enjoy big cruise liners with over 1000 passengers and where gambling casinos, discos, and the Las Vegas type of entertainment are featured.

It is, instead, for the thoughtful traveler, for the one who wishes to visit, but not despoil the native way of life. This is planned for the anthropologist, the photographer of wild life and rare birds, for the one who enjoys excellent lectures in the evening by experts knowledgeable about the region and the peoples to be visited the next day. There is no glitz.

A friend, Nancy Elsnab, the co-owner of Athenour Travel, recently went on the Orinoco River Exploration with Society Expeditions. The Orinoco River is located in Venezuela and the delta of the river is in a very remote part of this country. There were no roads in much of the area that they explored, but there were many branches of the river to navigate. These tributaries led them through thick jungle growth, and they were able to visit remote Indian villages.

Rare exotic birds flew overhead — macaws, parrots, red-billed toucans, hermit hummingbirds, and later, near Trinidad, hundreds of brilliant scarlet ibises coming home to roost at sunset in the mangroves. Monkeys chattered as they leapt from tree to tree. The "little howler monkey" was noisy and vociferous.

The group had adventures together they will never forget. They searched for alligators. They watched a bird devouring a piranha, and then fished for piranhas themselves. Later the guests ate these "mean little critters," these man-eating fish, as hors d'oeuvres!

They flew over Angel Falls, the highest one in the world at 3,212 feet. On that same day, they traveled from the 20th century world of flight in a modern plane back as if in a time machine to an ancient era. On the afternoon of the same day they explored the lagoon at Canaima National Park in dugout canoes.

The ship they sailed on, the *Society Explorer*, held a maximum of 96 passengers. All of the cabins were outside ones, so that everyone had a view through a porthole, or large picture windows if the more expensive category was booked.

The amenities are not overlooked on the ship. There is a medical center, a fitness center with a sauna, a library and a swimming pool. The passengers do not have to rush through their meals, so that another set of people can come in to dine, because there is single seating for meals in the spacious dining room with big view windows. If a flock of rare tropical birds fly past, you will not miss the colorful display while dining.

The three ships this company utilizes have shallow drafts, the very latest technology for navigating, and hulls which have been specially hardened so that the ships can explore ice-filled waters — a quality not needed on the Orinoco River!

The Zodiacs carried on board, developed by Jacques Cousteau for his explorations, are maneuverable and cannot be sunk. They carry up to fourteen passengers. With members of the crew on each Zodiac, guests are taken up narrow little tributaries and streams where no big ship could navigate.

In the Zodiacs, the passengers all wore life jackets and wore little back packs which held camera equipment. Their hands had to be free so that they could easily climb in and out of the Zodiac. To further protect their cameras they placed them in plastic bags. Nancy was able to successfully transport a video camera in this way and returned home with an amazing video she had taken herself.

The group explored the Rio Negro, a South American river deep in the jungle. They saw the strange "wedding of the waters." This phenomenon refers to the area where the deep brown-colored Rio Negro runs side by side with the cream-colored Amazon, but the two do not mix.

The participants visited an Indian village where the natives slept in hammocks in open huts. They lived in houses without walls, right on the water on raised platforms anchored on stilts.

Society Expeditions has an excellent policy of preserving the native way of life. They visit each little village perhaps only once in a year. These Indians did not want their pictures taken and were very superstitious. The travelers respected their wishes.

Gifts were given to the mayor or chief of the village. The gifts were soccer balls, basketballs and a gas-powered chain saw for the natives to use in clearing the land. They were given and accepted in the spirit of friendship. Nobody begged or bartered. Thus the native way of life remains unspoiled.

To book this adventure, see your travel agent who will also coordinate your flights, or —

Write or call:
> Society Expeditions Cruises, Inc.
> 3131 Elliott Ave., Suite 700
> Seattle, WA 98121
> (206) 285-9400

Cost: expensive, but the price is all inclusive, including the shore excursions. The cost varies according to the type of accommodations desired on the ship.

Fitness rating: moderate. Active older adults are encouraged to participate in every activity. In speaking to the expedition headquarters I was told of a very active 88-year-old gentleman who enthusiastically proved he was as fit as anyone on the voyage.

Wheelchair access: no

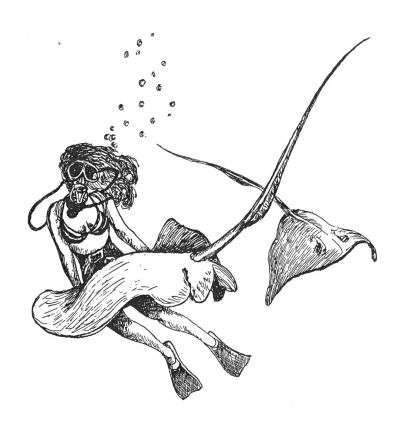

UNUSUAL ADVENTURES IN THE WESTERN CARIBBEAN

The Western Caribbean islands are among the most picturesque of the many islands in the Caribbean. Because they are nearer to the Atlantic coastlines of Florida and Mexico and are located in the western half of the Caribbean, they belong to that part of the world which some call the Western Caribbean.

At one time, many of these islands were known as the West Indies. There are more differences than similarities between these islands, however. On Haiti, the language is French; on other islands English is spoken. In other parts of the Caribbean, one can find the widespread influence of the Dutch, German, Portuguese, and Spanish.

GRAND CAYMAN

The adventures one can enjoy while visiting Grand Cayman in the Western Caribbean are vivid reminders that much of the world is comprised of water.

You can snorkel just offshore from George Town, or while swimming near the public beaches which dot the island. Parrots Landing, Grand Cayman, boasts of a watersports park where any visitor can snorkel without charge. Parrots Reef is here and the wreck of the *Anna Marie*. As a reef forms over old shipwrecks, the tropical fish make it their habitat, and many colorful beauties can be seen here, darting in and out of an old hull. One can rent or buy equipment as needed from the Dive Shop located at Parrots Landing just off of South Church Street, a mere 450 yards from George Town.

Grand Cayman is known all over the world as one of the finest areas for scuba divers. This is largely due to the efforts of the Cayman Watersports Operators Association (CWOA), because it has worked to protect and develop the natural resources found here. The Cayman Islands comprise a park, where all natural life in the sea is protected. Laws state that nothing can be removed from the water.

Boats which are owned by CWOA members are equipped with radios for emergencies, and the divers who belong to the organization know rescue techniques and frequently take part in simulated rescue practice operations. A well-equipped hospital and a recompression chamber are available.

If you are staying at a resort here, diving instruction is easily managed. After a few hours of training, shallow reef dives can transport you into the magical world below the sea.

Dive shops also rent underwater cameras with lights. If you are an avid photographer, there are courses offered for the techniques needed to successfully photograph underwater. Some diving trips specialize in photo sessions. You may only wish to record your own exploits while scuba diving. It is then possible to commission a video taping of your underseas adventure, or you may arrange to rent the equipment, and film your entire family exploring the many coral reefs.

STINGRAY CITY

Would you like to hug a stingray? This isn't your idea of romance? Then how about feeding one?

One of the most unusual diving areas in the world has been developed here. It is called Stingray City, and divers have the thrill of feeding and touching or hugging a stingray. Here the stingrays have been almost tamed by man, and they will swim up and eat bread out of a diver's hand.

A friend who has dived here said, "The stingrays are like big puppy dogs. They nudged me and followed me everywhere."

At least 28 stingrays have learned that people, in this one area, are friends to be trusted and a source of food. Normally shy, these great grey creatures might playfully nip the hand that feeds them, so wearing gloves is recommended. My friend also ran her hand on their underbelly, and she said that area is very smooth and soft. She then put her gloves back on before feeding them more food. Wouldn't you?

Write or call:
> Fisheye
> Trafalgar Place
> West Bay Road
> P.O. Box 2123
> Grand Cayman, B.W. I.
> (809) 947-4209

Cost: inexpensive (in 1990) for a Stingray City dive if you are already an accomplished and certified diver. Moderate if you wish an edited video tape of your dive, accompanied by music. Inexpensive to rent a 35 mm underwater camera for half a day.   It is expensive for the novice diver course — best to have the training in your home area.

Fitness rating: moderate; ability to swim a plus.

Scuba Diving "High"

While waiting for my plane in Honolulu recently in the international lounge, I overheard two middle-aged women talking excitedly. One of them had silver hair and both were slim and bronzed from the sun.

"I don't know why I didn't try it years ago."

"I don't either. Nothing I've ever done has given me more of a thrill."

I sauntered over and visited with them. Their excitement bubbled over and was infectious. They had both spent a week in Fiji learning to scuba dive and both of them were very eager for their next vacation so that they could experience that "high" down in the depths of the sea again.

I personally believe this sport can be mastered by any age group as long as one possesses courage, common sense, and good lungs. Learn and be guided by a reputable diver, and away you go! This is definitely a sport to be shared. Always go with a "buddy."

If, however, you do not wish to scuba dive and have only a limited time on Grand Cayman, there are at least three other adventures you could embark upon.

WORLD'S LARGEST GLASS BOTTOM BOAT

If you or your offspring have had a small aquarium in your home, you are well aware of how hypnotizing the fish swimming about can be. If you tried to preserve tropical fish in a salt water tank, you will undoubtedly remember how difficult it was to keep these delicate fish alive and well, and how difficult it was to clean out the tank.

On a glass bottom boat, you are a guest. You just enjoy watching the lively fish beneath you and you don't have to clean a thing. Stretched out before your eyes is the biggest aquarium you'll ever see.

The *Cayman Mermaid* is hailed as the "World's Largest Glass Bottom Boat." Day trips and evening trips are scheduled, and in the evening the water is illuminated so that you can view red groupers, Naussau groupers, and some of the other fish which are liveliest at night.

This boat serves cocktails aboard and there is one stop at a beach near a reef for those who wish to snorkel. For nonswimmers who prefer to stay aboard there are the usual amenities, and as the ship cruises back to George Town there is dancing on board to a native band. Popular with crowds from the occasional cruise ship which comes into port here, there is even a limbo demonstration on board.

In the limbo, the native dancer punishes his or her body by bending backwards further and further until the back of the head almost touches the floor, as the body gyrates under a pole which is lowered after each successful time the dancer goes under it without grazing the pole. It looks painful and impossible, but the performer comes out of these contortions with an enormous smile.

Write or call:
> Cayman Mermaid
> Royal Palms Beach
> George Town, Grand Cayman, B.W. I.
> (809) 947-5132

Cost: inexpensive for a three-hour tour, including the entertainment

Fitness rating: easy

SUB-SEA EXPLORER

For an unusual voyage, try the *Sub-Sea Explorer.* I experienced this recently and it gave me the illusion of being underwater. An unimposing-looking sea craft on the water's surface, it still gives "land lubbers" a tremendous thrill. We were invited to go down a flight of steps and then sat two abreast. My companion happened to be a museum director, traveling with his wife and daughter. They took a keen delight in every wonder, just as I did. A narrator described the reef and identified the many brilliant fish which we could see.

On the lower level there were windows instead of walls on both sides of us and our view was unobstructed. The one-inch-thick glass is of the same thickness as that used on airplanes. This glass magnified everything we saw, making it all appear 25 percent larger and 25 percent closer. We really felt that the craft was almost touching the sharp formations of the coral reef because of this phenomenon. Our guide had one warning for us as we gazed out.

"Please don't open the windows!"

The first reef we approached is termed Killer Reef or Cheeseburger Reef by the natives, and it is just offshore. A school of barracudas swam past, probably at least 50 or 60 of them — immature barracudas about a third the size of adult ones. Nassau groupers with brown and white stripes were larger than some of the tiny yellowhead wrasse. The groupers seemed to stay closer to the ocean's floor and are usually more active at night. Since they feed on other fish I was glad it was their inactive period.

We viewed a long four-and-a-half-foot silver-hued fish called a turbot which is often mistaken for a shark. A big school of brilliant blue tangs came in close as the diver fed them bread crumbs. At one point, so many fish of such varied colors surrounded our diver that he was invisible to us. Only the bubbles of air from his tank marked his location. I was suddenly reminded of the thousands of pigeons in Piazzo San Marco in Venice. Birds and fish both seem to know how to find a free hand-out.

The deep blue angelfish with the yellow eye, and the exquisite blue-green queen angelfish are a common sight here and follow divers who offer them cheese. Oceanic trigger fish are numerous.

Many shipwrecks are in this region — hence the nickname Killer Reef. We glided over the wreck of a freighter, the *Cali*, which sank in 1936. All men were saved, but the cargo of rice and grain expanded as it became wet, and the ship went down quickly. Today, coral is beginning to form over the submerged hull and it will be another reef in time, but coral is slow growing and fragile. It can take 20 years for one inch of coral to develop.

As we went over the Arizona reef, we learned it was a nickname for an "infant reef," one just beginning to form. The one-celled organisms are still alive. Because the young coral resembles cactus plants in the sand, an airline pilot visiting here said it reminded him of Arizona, and that became its name.

Write:
Sub Sea Explorer
Royal Palms Beach
George Town, Grand Cayman, B.W. I.
Cost: inexpensive
Fitness rating: easy

ATLANTIS SUBMARINE

Have you ever wondered what it would be like to go down into the ocean's depths in a submarine? A short voyage on the spectacular *Atlantis Submarine* costs slightly more than double the price of a Sub-Sea Explorer adventure. This is the world's first submarine created exclusively for people who wish to see what fascinates the scuba diver. It can hold a maximum of 28 passengers, who are taken to Grand Cayman's outer reef where the sub descends to a depth of 150 feet. There is an informative lecture while the passengers view the marine life from portholes. As you glide past unusual sponge gardens and view schools of colorful tropical fish, you may also enjoy complete comfort.

Children from 4 to 12 years old are charged half price, so if you are vacationing with grand-children, this tour might be ideal. While appropriate for all ages, this trip is not for those who suffer from claustrophobia. The *Atlantis Submarine* trip is also available in Honolulu and Kona. I have a good friend who treated her daughter and grand-daughter to this excursion, and for her it was the best treat of anything that they did in a ten-day period while exploring the Western Caribbean.

Write or call:
    Atlantis Submarine
    South Church Street
    Grand Cayman, B.W. I.
    (809) 949-8383
Cost: inexpensive; half-price for children from 4 to 12 years
Fitness rating:

The Atlantis Submarine is also available in Hawaii, from Honolulu or off the coast of Kona.

RESEARCH SUBMERSIBLES, LTD.

The third way to explore these waters and not get your feet wet is the most unusual and the most costly. For about $100 at this writing, you can go diving in the *Research Submersibles, Ltd.* This submarine can dive down to 800 feet and holds only two passengers and a professional pilot-guide per dive. Because you can dive to such a depth, you will view uncommon life forms not seen closer to the water's surface.

Nor are all the wonders wrought by nature. The man-made ship, the *Kirk Pride,* is a 500-ton freighter that sank in 1975. For ten years its whereaaabouts was a mystery, but a pilot in a research submarine finally located it. Since it lies on a ledge at a depth of 780 feet, it has the distinction of being one of the world's deepest wrecks. Only those who venture out in the *Research Submersible* can see this.

Because of the lights of this submarine, flash attachments on your camera are not needed, and passengers can take as many underwater pictures as they wish with their own camera equipment.

Once more, this trip is not recommended for anyone who is claustophobic or who does not fancy being enclosed in small quarters, but if you wish to rub noses with a hogfish or a stoplight parrotfish through a protective layer of glass, this may be the perfect adventure for you.

Write or call:
      Research Submersibles, Ltd.
      North Church Street
      George Town, Grand Cayman, B.W. I.
      (809) 949-8296
Cost: expensive
Fitness rating: easy

A VISIT TO HELL

If you do not wish to leave the land, Grand Cayman is the one place where you can go to Hell, survive the experience, and live to tell others of your adventure.

Hell is situated on the west end of Grand Cayman Island, very near the Cayman Turtle Farm. You can rent a car for a nominal fee in George Town or join a tour which will combine the two destinations. If you rent a car, or engage a taxi as a group, drive along Seven Mile Beach, stop for snorkeling and a glorious swim, and proceed along the road until you reach the turtle farm.

The Cayman Turtle Farm claims to be the only one of its kind in the world. It is bringing the sea turtle back from the brink of extinction. Sea turtles are bred and raised here. Once hunted for food and for its shell, the population is now increasing. While some are later sold for food, a certain percentage have to be returned to the sea each year and the operation is a success.

At the turtle farm you may be lucky enough to see a small turtle emerge from its egg. The tiny newborn turtle, perfectly formed, can weigh as little as six ounces. The biggest of the sea turtles can weigh a hefty 600 pounds. Snorkelers commonly see large healthy sea turtles in the wild near here, where they are protected while living out their lives in the warm waters surrounding Grand Cayman.

Hell is very near to this breeding turtle farm and is located on Spanish Bay. The extraordinary rock formations here are the reason for the name. Formed out of limestone, the shapes are surreal and at night might be quite terrifying. The small town, named a century ago, does a brisk business today in selling postcards for its visitors from Hell to mail to destinations all over the world.

A day spent snorkeling or swimming, touring the Cayman Turtle Farm, and visiting Hell would be suitable for all ages, a delight for grandparents and their grandchildren, and would be nominal in cost. Who knows? After seeing those strange and surreal forms of limestone, your grandchildren might turn out to be angels for the rest of your vacation.

Write or call:
> Cayman Turtle Farm
> Box 645
> West Bay, Grand Cayman B.W. I.
> (809) 949-3894

Cost: inexpensive
Fitness rating: easy

AN INTERLUDE IN JAMAICA:
A RIDE IN A TRACTOR-PULLED JITNEY

Also located in the West Indies, Jamaica is well worth a visit. Here the language is again English, but a strongly accented one with a beautiful lilt. The half-day tour to the Brimmer Hall Estate is unusual because while there, the visitor is pulled along behind a farm tractor in a wagon-like rig or jitney that holds about 20 people, sitting back to back, with poles for the passengers to clutch.

It is fun to ask yourself how many different ways you have traveled in your lifetime — by horse, camel, airplane, balloon, ship, etc. Although I've ridden on farm tractors, I've never been in a conveyance pulled by one. As a mode of transportation, its virtue lies in being slow enough to let the passengers smell the flowers. Nor does it have to remain on paved roads. Like the tractor or a jeep, it can go across fields and up small hills.

We not only saw tiny wild flowers, but stopped frequently to examine fields of growing crops, like pineapple in all its many stages. We looked at coffee beans, coconut trees, and cocoa. Examining the cocoa bean which is harvested here, we found that inside the bean many pods are surrounded by a gelatinous white substance. Each of us sampled one pod and were rewarded with a bitter lemony taste that puckered up our mouths and had no resemblance to cocoa.

The banana trees were fascinating because one can also see all of the stages of growth in a single visit. Our guide picked a tiny cluster. Perhaps 50 future bananas clung together in a small fist-sized sphere, each one a tiny green ribbon no larger than a kernel of rice.

The Brimmer Hall Plantation is in the vicinity of Port Maria, Jamaica and comprises about 2,000 acres. The house on the estate was built in the 18th century. Hand-crafted then by native slaves, the ceilings, windows and floors were fashioned out of indigenous hardwoods. The furniture is primarily of dark mahogany, and although this home does not compare to the magnificance of the southern plantations, it looks as though the owners had a very comfortable life.

Today the old horse stables have been turned into a series of shops featuring native wood sculptures, the ubiquitous T-shirts, dresses, dashikis (a woman's wrap-around cloth) and world-famous Jamaican rum. A note of caution. If you purchase a wooden hand-carved sculpture, either give it to your worst enemy, the boss who fired you last year, or place it in the freezer for at least 24 hours. Termites are abundant in Jamaica.

Visitors are welcome to swim in the pool here and use the changing rooms. The pool area is surrounded by magnificent beds of roses and lilies, and the trellises are covered with deep purple bougainvillea. From a vantage point here, a gazebo-like structure, there are beautiful vistas as the land drops away.

On the route out from Ocho Rios to the plantation, one sees the former home of Ian Fleming, who created the character of James Bond, and many other estates belonging to celebrities, including Sir Noel Coward. One also sees the devastation caused recently by Hurrican Gilbert. An entire area of housing has only the foundations left. Slowly, that area is coming alive again, and structures are rising.

It is a sobering reminder of nature's fury and I would recommend staying away from the Caribbean during the hurricane season of late August,

September, and early October. If you don't mind taking the risk, however, that is the time of year for the greatest financial bargains in vacation rentals.

As you return by a different, more mountainous route from the tour of the plantation, you pass small native villages, and as you approach Ocho Rios you can see a big estate where one of the James Bond films was produced.

If one is on the longer tour of this island, one is then taken to visit famous Dunn's River Falls. Try to take some time here. Do not sign on with a tour which only promises you a photo stop. One needs to savor this experience and if you want to get in on the thrill of climbing up the waterfall as the water meanders down over rocks and boulders in a very gradual descent, allow at least an hour or two.

If you are staying several days in Jamaica, drive or take a taxi to Dunn's River Falls and spend a morning or an afternoon here. The cost is nominal for a native guide to take you on the exciting climb. Because you are in the water, wear a swimsuit and tennis shoes — zoris might be lost in the water. Avoid exploring the falls on the days that a major cruise ship docks in Ocho Rios.

I had always wanted to see this area and have gazed at photos of it for years, which look pristine and full of lush beauty and vegetation. I have a friend who was fortunate enough to explore the falls in May when she and her sister were the only ones in the river with the native guide.

I saw it, unfortunately, when two giant cruise ships were in port, and the guides were leading a long string of humanity which all but obliterated the beauty. Everyone was laughing and enjoying himself and it is such a gradual climb that all ages from three to seventy seemed to be involved. But who wants to enjoy nature with a cast of thousands?

Barbecued food can be purchased here and many natives are selling handicrafts ranging from woven baskets to those wooden sculptures which need freezing. Not even the shopper in your family needs to feel excluded from enjoying this area.

Write or call:
> Brimmer Hall Estate
> Plantation Tour
> Jamaica, B.W. I.
> (809) 994-2309

Cost: inexpensive
Fitness rating: moderate for climbing the falls, easy for the tour to the Brimmer Hall Estate

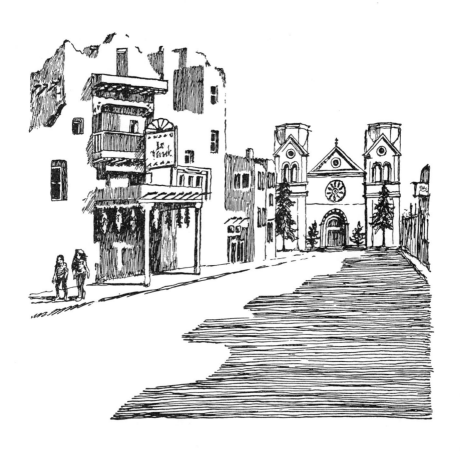

NEW MEXICO ADVENTURES

BANDELIER NATIONAL PARK

Not far out of Santa Fe, New Mexico, an unusual travel adventure awaits the visitor. Have you ever wanted to explore caves which were inhabited by man hundreds of years ago? Have you ever wondered how the native Anasazi Indians managed to live in caves which are high up on the face of cliffs? By visiting Bandelier National Park, ten miles out of Los Alamos, where the atomic bomb was first created, one travels back in time at least 500 years.

The Indians thrived in this environment. Today the park has over 72 miles of trails to explore. Backpackers can hike in and camp, but must stay on the trail. One can explore the region on horseback and campfires are permitted in most areas. Campers cannot, however, stay adjacent to the famous archeological sites which have been uncovered.

Most visitors are less adventurous and elect to take a tour which originates in Santa Fe. This tour just covers the highlights of Bandelier National Park, but, accompanied by a naturalist/guide, one can learn much about the Indians' way of life. Although the park now boasts 32,737 acres, the first-time visitor may be content to view the caves by clambering up the ladders which lead to some of the more accessible caves.

As you climb the trails, from a distance you spot dark openings in the cliffs — openings which are actually caves. Centuries ago, wind and water erosion created small openings, and the Indians who came later worked to enlarge these holes to form the caves which became their homes. These caves, as you explore them, sheltered the Anasazi from the elements — from rain, sleet, hail storms, and lightning, and from intense cold and searing heat.

Women should wear slacks or shorts to this national park. I made the mistake of wearing a dress and then was too modest to climb the ladders and explore the tempting caves. Children had a great time scampering up to the caves and peaking in.

The Anasazi lived in these canyons between 1100 A.D. and 1600 A.D. It is thought that droughts may have forced them to move into villages nearer to the Rio Grande River. The soil may no longer have been fertile, drinking water difficult to find and firewood depleted.

Whatever the reason for the mass exodus, the area today fascinates the visitor. The stone cliffs of pink and white look tall and inhospitable. It seems unbelievable that mankind existed here for centuries.

To explore the more remote back country, one must secure a permit which is available from the Visitor Center. In order to camp overnight, a permit is also required.

For the day visitor, wheelchairs are available at the Visitor Center. From a wheelchair, a person who might have a difficult time exploring this area can tour the Tyounyi ruins which are quite close, and then traverse the nature trail which is on the valley floor, surrounded by towering cliffs.

Archaeologists have recorded about 1,260 sites in Bandelier National Park. At least 350 recorded rooms have been found in the Yapashi area. Evidence has been uncovered which indicates that nomadic people were here in this region from 1 A.D.

A short tour to Bandelier National Park to see the cliff dwellings can be arranged through Santa Fe Detours.

Call:
> Santa Fe Detours
> (800) DETOURS

Cost: moderate; half price for children ages 5 to 12. Many family groups enjoy this tour, and it would be a good one for grandparents and their grandchildren.
Fitness rating: minimal to strenuous
Wheelchair access: yes, for the shorter tour

THE SHRINE OF THE STONE LIONS

A two-day hike is suggested if the backpacker wishes to visit the Shrine of the Stone Lions. To get here, one must be in good health and acclimated to the 7,000 foot elevation. Purchase or bring with you a topographic map of the region and discuss your plans with a park ranger. If you don't return when expected, a search party will be organized to rescue you. It is, of course, best for one to hike with a good friend or in a small compatible group.

To reach the shrine, count on twelve miles of good hiking, round trip. As one ascends the "Grand Staircase," he climbs hundreds of steps hewn out of rock. The Alamo Canyon is 500 feet deep and has steep cliffs. A mile away the hiker comes upon Yapashi, the ruins where archaeologists are still discovering rooms and kivas, the sites where people gathered for their religious ceremonies.

Beyond Yapashi in a forest of pinon trees are the two crouching mountain lions carved out of sandstone. Large boulders stand like tall sentries guarding this site from interlopers. Although now damaged by erosion, often antlers and food offerings are placed near the lions, because for our native Americans, it is a shrine.

Exercise common sense on hikes in this region. Stay on the trail, do not befriend the wild creatures which might carry bubonic plague, and do not drink the water without preparing it carefully. The water here is all contaminated with giardia, a tiny organism which causes diarrhea and can make one feel very uncomfortable.

If a thunderstorm strikes, move off the higher mesa areas and head towards the lower elevations. Lightning can be a danger here.

For a longer backpacking adventure, take your own car and gear, or fly into Albuquerque, rent a car and drive up to the national park. It is common to see a hiker with a backpack entering a plane.

A useful guide for hiking in this park is *Guide to Bandelier National Monument* by Dorothy Hoard. Published by Los Alamos Historical Society, it contains useful maps and history of the region. ($5.95)

Write:
   Bandelier National Monument Visitor Center
   Bandelier National Park, NM 87544
Cost: inexpensive
Fitness rating: moderate to strenuous. Explore at your own pace.
Wheelchair access: no

CUMBRES AND TOLTEC SCENIC RAILROAD
While still exploring New Mexico, you might want a more civilized adventure, particularly if you are a

railroad enthusiast.

Instead of leaping back centuries in time, the Cumbres and Toltec Scenic Railroad takes the traveler back about 100 years. This train operated in 1880 and into the early part of the 20th century, and was originally designed to serve the remote mining camps located in the San Juan Mountains.

Experience the excitement of traveling 64 miles on this narrow-gauge steam train which has daily excursions. As the train takes you down into valleys and up near the mountain peaks of the Rockies, you will hear the whistle echo in the tunnels, and see the hissing steam as the train rounds the bends in the mountains. The odor of coal smoke, pungent and acrid, will mingle in the air with the scent of pines and aspen.

The track is laid through beautiful gorges, dark tunnels and over trestles. It crests at the 10,015 foot Cumbres Pass. Lucius Beebe termed this ride, "The most awesomely spectacular example of mountain railroading in North America." Today it is a Registered National Historic Site and is owned by the states of New Mexico and Colorado.

The sightseeing car is open to the elements, but on the rest of the coaches, windows can be closed if it rains or turns cold. The weather in the summer can be warm, but it is unpredictable. There is no heater on the train, so wear the "layered look." Take jackets and sweaters and peel them off when you are down on the valley floor.

The train leaves daily from either Chama, New Mexico, or Antonito, Colorado, and since there is no public transportation, you must drive to Chama — 107 miles from Santa Fe, New Mexico — or to Antonito.

The train stops in Osier in the middle of the day and passengers buy a hot lunch there or bring their own picnic.

There are certain cars which are equipped with a wheelchair lift. Advise the reservations clerk of this need when booking the trip and reserve this at least seven days prior to travel.

You may reserve space with either credit cards (Visa or Mastercard) or with a check. Seniors are entitled to a 10% discount, but it must be requested when booked. This is a seasonal train. The schedule shows daily runs from the end of May until the middle of October. Once the snow pack settles in, the track may be inaccessible for the winter months.

Write or call:
Cumbres and Toltec Scenic Railroad
P.O. Box 789
Chama, NM 87520
(505) 756-2151
Cost: inexpensive
Fitness rating: easy
Wheelchair access: yes

THE SANTA FE OPERA

While in the area of Santa Fe in the summer, try to arrange to see an opera. This takes advance planning because the season is frequently sold out. It is a fascinating combination, to view the ancient Indian pueblos or to explore Bandelier National Park by day, and then in the evening, as darkness falls, to hear a magnificent, rarely performed opera out under the stars. If you would like to hear several operas in the week that you are visiting here, read on!

"I have two tickets to sell if you wish them," I said to the distinguished looking gentleman and his wife.

He was delighted to purchase the tickets to Mozart's *Cosi Fan Tutte.* The box office was sold out and only standing room was left. As we talked, I learned he was a violinist and an eye surgeon. His interesting accent proved to be Hungarian, so I placed him near a woman in our group who was also of Hungarian birth.

It turned out that the couple was seated directly in front of me, so we talked of playing chamber music and of our favorite operas.

The magic of Mozart commenced and my entire group of 25 opera lovers became engrossed in the music and the absurd tale of two men, very much in love, testing the fidelity of their ladies.

The night grew colder, the wind began to blow, and at the first intermission, sweaters and coats or jackets were added. No longer did we look like an elegant theater crowd dressed for a night at the opera. Lightning flashed in the sky. We were under a protective roof, but the sides and certain sections were open to the dramatic electric storm.

By the second intermission I was shivering. A woman seated next to me whispered, "I have a couple of garbage bags with me. Would you like one?"

Forgetting all efforts to impress our distinguished visitors, I happily accepted. Offering to share my treasure with a lady who was also shivering, we huddled together, our legs encased in the dark ugly plastic bag pulled up to our waists.

Toasty and warm now, we lost ourselves in the last act, joking afterwards about being two bag ladies.

While I was still standing in the bag afterwards, the courtly gentleman kissed my Hungarian friend's hand and my own — a touching continental gesture. It was certainly my first kiss while standing in a garbage bag!

To arrange tickets for the Santa Fe Opera —

Call:
    Santa Fe Opera Box Office
    (505) 982-3855
Cost: expensive
Fitness rating: easy
Wheelchair access: yes

Don't overlook your local college or junior college for tours to hear magnificent concerts and operas or to visit galleries and museums.

I have been organizing educational tours for Chabot College, located in Hayward, California for several years. Our prices are kept low because we usually stay in student dormitories during the summer season when the students are on vacation. For those on a budget this helps considerably. The tour price includes breakfast and dinner daily, and stimulating lectures each day from our college instructor, transportation and tours to nearby Indian pueblos, at least four opera tickets, a day in Taos, and round trip air transportation from the Oakland Airport. Thus far we have been lucky with the weather. The night described above has been our only rainy cold night in seeing ten operas.

SEE SANTA FE

Santa Fe is a very interesting destination in its own right. Planned in Spain in the early 17th century, it was settled by colonists from Spain. The early style of architecture is preserved and there are strict building codes, so that the unique character of its buildings will not be destroyed by high-rise development.

The far-sighted plans put into effect in 1957 state that only the Spanish-Pueblo or territorial style of architecture may be used in the historic portions of Santa Fe, and no building can be more that five stories high. As the visitor walks through the areas of this unique capital, his eyes feast on the beauty of the buildings.

After World War ll, the city fathers declared that they did not want a big airport built nearby, and even the train stops several miles out of town in the middle of "nowhere," according to one brochure.

It has thus remained a historical gem set apart from its modern neighbor, Albuquerque, 65 miles to the southwest. Santa Fe is the nation's only state capitol that has no modern commercial airport. For a wealthy few and for emergencies there is a small airport outside of town, but no modern jets or gigantic planes arrive and take off. Mesa Airlines, with its Beechcrafts and Cessnas, carry between four and nineteen passengers from Denver, Albuquerque and Taos, but most prefer ground transportation.

Because of this isolation from the noise and bustle of trains and planes, and because of its strict building codes, it reminds one of Taxco in Mexico — another historical jewel.

Transportation is easily arranged from Albuquerque with "Shuttlejack" or Santa Fe Detours. Transportation to the center of Santa Fe from the train station some eight or nine miles away can also be prearranged. In addition, of course, cars can be rented at the Albuquerque Airport, and families and friends can then drive themselves to Santa Fe.

One of the most delightful ways to explore Santa Fe is with a walking tour of the older historic portions of the city. If possible, book it with Waite Thompson, the author of *The Santa Fe Guide.* His book is an excellent guide, and his infectious sense of humor is interlaced with history and anecdotes which make it an experience well worth leaving the protective cocoon of your car or bus to hear. His walks depart daily from the La Fonda Hotel lobby at 9:30 A.M. and at 1:30 P.M. The three-and-a-half-mile stroll lasts for approximately two and a half hours, and the cost is minimal. If a child under age 14 is accompanied by an adult there is no charge.

Anyone in good health would thoroughly enjoy this walk, but if you have just arrived in Santa Fe and are not acclimatized yet to its 7000+ foot altitude or have high blood pressure, this may not be the best way for you to explore Santa Fe. Many walk part of the way, enjoying Thompson's talk thoroughly, and drop out discreetly when they become tired.

I have planned our college tours to include four or five operas given by the Santa Fe Opera, now enjoying its 34th season. Because of the climate in Santa Fe, the season is a short one and the opera lover needs to order tickets well in advance. The season commences on the last weekend in June and runs until the last Saturday night in August. Productions are given six nights a week with no performances on Sundays.

The operas are lavishly staged, the costumes are magnificent and the musical standards are very high. Conceived by General Director John Crosby many years ago, it is now recognized the world over and offers productions which rival those given in any first class opera house. It is also known for giving each year a new American or world premier. With the beauty of the natural setting and the superb voices of singers like Marilyn Horne, it is easy to understand why the Santa Fe Opera has built up a loyal following.

If you are planning your own trip, single opera tickets are quite expensive and must be ordered in advance. Hotels and motels range from reasonable to expensive, but food and excellent dining at many fine retaurants is less expensive than in major American cities.

If you live in the San Francisco Bay Region, for an all-inclusive tour, including air and optional college credit —

Write or call:

    Chabot College
    Office of Community Development
    25555 Hesperian Blvd.
    Hayward, California 94545
    (415) 786-6600 or my office: (415) 846-8069

Cost: inexpensive, until one adds the operas; then cost is moderate

Fitness rating: minimal

Wheelchair access: yes, at the opera, but not as yet in the college dorm where the college tour stays.

If you live far from the San Francisco Bay Region, to receive, free of charge, a 65-page colored book and guide —

Write or call:

    Santa Fe Convention and Visitors Center
    P.O. Box 909
    Santa Fe, NM 87504-0909
    (800) 777-2489

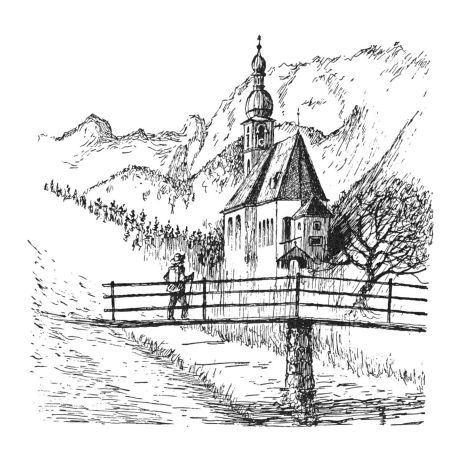

WALKING TOURS IN EUROPE

A TALE OF THREE COUNTRIES

Have you ever seen a man with a power mower cutting the grass on the roof of his sod house? My friends, Ariel and Bob, were startled when they saw just that in Chamonix, France. Sod roofs have been around for centuries and are now very expensive to maintain, but a 20th century power mower is an incongruous sight atop a roof which may date back to the middle ages! If you embark on a walking tour in Europe or the British Isles, this is the type of detail you may see.

When you whiz by an idyllic scene on a tour bus, you are unable to tarry in one area long enough to talk with the local inhabitants, identify an unusual wild flower or bird, or just satisfy your curiosity.

Walking is beneficial for our health, and for those of you with a zest for adventure and healthy exercise, and the time to indulge yourself, a walking tour may be the answer.

Ariel and Bob Witbeck of Danville, California recently joined the University of California Alumni Association on a walking tour through portions of Switzerland, France and Italy. They enjoyed themselves with a compatible group which ranged in age from the late 40s to an 82-year-old retired professor. Ariel assured me that the retired professor was always the first one to complete the hike and the first one up in the morning. He seemed filled with more energy than some who were 30 years younger.

They stayed three or four nights in each hotel and hiked out from that base. This was not exactly roughing it, for they never unrolled their sleeping bags under the stars. Each night they returned to hot showers or baths, a good dinner and the warmth and comfort of a good bed. They only had to hike with their day's supplies, not with a mammoth backpack.

Making their lunches from the buffet breakfast served in the hotel was done with the hotel's blessing. Have you ever spied the frugal tourist secretly stowing away a breakfast roll spread with jam or cheese for his free lunch, while others of us paid top dollar for a big hot European meal? I have.

But on this tour, by prior arrangement and payment, the waiters brought out extra rolls, cheeses and cold cuts for this purpose. Each hiker then carried his own lunch and a canteen of water. The hotels even furnished ice water for the canteens.

Seven miles was the greatest distance walked. They began their walking tour in Chamonix after flying into the Geneva Airport. A chartered motorcoach transported them to their hotel in Chamonix. From here they could view the "roof of Europe," as Mont Blanc is called.

One of the highlights was visiting the Mer De Glace after a ridge walk along the Grand Balcon Nord to Montenvers at 6,275 feet. A cable car took the walkers to the famous Mer de Glace, a glacier which is snow-covered all year around. Here they saw huge ice sculptures, one entire living room carved in ice, and an ice statue of a bear which the Cal alumni enjoyed, as the bear is their mascot.

From Chamonix they piled into a bus and traveled through the tunnel between Switzerland and Italy to Stresa, Italy and later to Sirmione, a resort which is clustered around Scalinger's Castle, built in the 13th century. In their hotel they could take advantage of thermal hot tubs.

Ariel said that it was the best of both worlds — healthy exercise each day and comfort every night with the hotels often offering jacuzzis or hot baths for aching muscles, as well as delicious dinners. To the delight of the women, they could shed their jeans, hiking clothes, and boots, and dress informally for dinner.

Their particular walking tour took them also to Verona, the medieval city made famous by Romeo and Juliet, where the participants walked around the older sections on foot. This is the best way to view many a European city in its preserved medieval sections.

They also hiked in the Dolomites at approximately 4,055 feet and ended their tour in Ortisei, where they walked, after catching a chairlift to Raschotz at 6,921 feet. As their Norwegian guide, Arne said, "We will walk a little up and a little down." This would make all the hikers, not as accustomed to the rugged terrain as he was, groan in protest, but they glowed with personal satisfaction after the hike.

A note of caution: This tour would not be good for those of you who can not adjust to heights near 7,000 feet or who have high blood pressure. There are, however, delightful walking tours in England in the Lake Country, which are low in altitude, in Scotland, and in other parts of Europe which are closer to sea level.

While this alumni tour was expensive with all the

amenities and two guides, other walking tours are inexpensive if the hikers camp out under the stars or stay in small huts where they prepare their own meals.

Write or call:

Mountain Travel
1398 Solano Avenue
Albany, CA 94706
(415) 527-8100

Cost: expensive

Fitness rating: strenuous, unless you are a daily walker or jogger

Wheelchair access: no

OTHER WALKING TOURS:
THE BRITISH ISLES

"To test the waters" to see if a walking tour is right for you, you might arrange for a short weekend or for a few days with a company in the British Isles which has been arranging walking vacations for twelve years. The company is called English Wanderer. It appears that their location is also the headquarters for Scottish Wanderer, Crwdryn Cymreig (Welsh Wanderer), and Irish Roamer.

A friend, Judy Ticehurst, arranged her flights in the United States, wrote to England for her walking tour, arrived a few days early so that she could explore the town of Ticehurst in England (where she believed her ancestors had lived), and then joined a walking tour in Hampshire. The groups stayed in the Ashburn Hotel with private baths and an outdoor pool, so again she wasn't roughing it. They walked in the New Forest, saw roe deer and New Forest ponies, walked across open heaths along Hampton Ridge and formed many new friends.

This company grades its tours in the following manner:

D is easy	—	8 - 11 miles a day
C is fairly easy	—	9 - 12 miles a day
C+ is moderate	—	9 - 14 miles a day

Boots are needed for the C+ tour and this one carries the additional warning: "Some longer and steeper ascents are involved so you should be in good shape."

A weekend walking tour in East Sussex has an added flavor. The guests stay in a former smuggler's home. Weekend rates in low season here are reasonable.

Write or call:
English Wanderer
13 Wellington Court, Spencer's Wood
Reading, RG7 1BN, England
44 -734-882515
Cost: inexpensive
Fitness rating: moderate for D and C, strenuous for C+
Wheelchair access: no

For more about walking tours, read on.

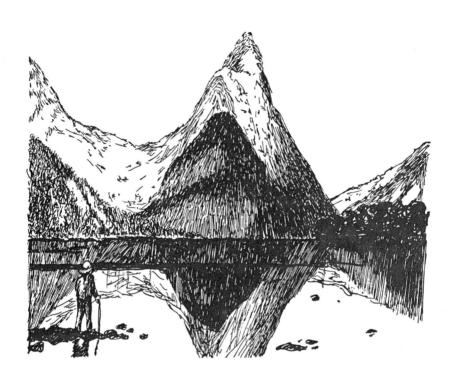

BEAUTIFUL NEW ZEALAND

THE MILFORD TRACK: ONE OF THE MOST FAMOUS OF ALL WALKING TOURS

The Milford Track in New Zealand has had a wide appeal to my husband and me for years. His mother was a Mackinnon who was born in Scotland. It was Quinton Mackinnon who discovered the pass in the Milford Sound area which made it possible to trek in and out of there. It bears his name still today —

Mackinnon Pass.

My husband Bill's uncle first went on the Milford Trek or Track when he was in his late 60s. When we saw his slides, his enthusiasm was contagious. Our son began saving his money and about eight years ago he signed up for the Milford Track.

He has never returned to live in California. Instead, we have made five trips "down under." I therefore have a bittersweet relationship with this area of great scenic beauty and spectacular contrasts. Rudyard Kipling called the Milford Sound the "eighth wonder of the world."

That the trek can be enjoyed by any age is amazing, but at the present time, it is restricted to those between the ages of 10 and 70. If a 70-year-old can prove he or she is in excellent health, then the upper age limit is waived, but small children are not allowed because of the danger of flash floods. It is also a seasonable hike, from early November to the middle of April. It is graded as an easy walk, although many miles a day are covered.

The Milford Track, or walk, from Te Anau Hotel to the Milford Sound is through some of the most beautiful countryside to be found anywhere. It is also an adventure. You should try to carry no more than twelve pounds, and should have a rain coat with you. It is a walk through glades of lush tree ferns made green because rain falls here all year long.

At your first bunkhouse, where the men sleep in

one and the women in another, you are provided with comforters, towels, a pillow and a cotton sleeping bag. The light-weight cotton sleeping bag and matching pillowcase you carry with you the rest of the trek, but you leave the heavy comforter and pillow behind. Each night you are issued a fresh towel.

Bird life seen along the Milford Track can include the southern crested grebe and the very rare, flightless takahe, which has red feet and bill, and iridescent blue-green feathers. It is exciting for Americans to walk along the trail and suddenly encounter two or three fiordland crested penguins waddling towards them, a frequent occurrence as one nears the sound. Our son saw the flightless kakapo one evening, for this fellow is nocturnal. His colorings are yellow-green and he resembles a ground parrot. Other animals to be seen here are red deer, wild pig, and *wapiti*, the native term for elk.

If you wish to have this wonderful adventure, it can be arranged through your travel agent, and should be booked well in advance.

If you have patience and can book a year in advance, you can arrange an independent reservation. Only 24 people can be scheduled each day of the season. They must travel in one direction only from Te Anau to the Milford Sound, and abide by the rules of the Track, but the cost is far less.

Write:

> Tourist Hotel Corporation
> P.O. Box 185
> Te Anau, New Zealand

Cost: for the five day, four night trek — moderate for adults, inexpensive for children. For an independent reservation, cost is inexpensive.
Fitness rating: moderate.

BY LAND AND BY SEA:
ANOTHER WAY TO EXPLORE THE SOUND

Sound here means fiord and the Milford Sound once was a valley surrounded by glaciers. The valley is now below sea level and as the ice melted, the valley became flooded. If you wish, there are day trips which can be arranged. Either drive in your rental car or take the bus tour out of Queenstown, and then enjoy a cruise on the Milford Sound. Here you are very apt to see fur seals. The *MV Milford Haven* cruises around the sound and out to the Tasman Sea.

While on this boat, try not to spend too much time over lunch because you might miss the magnificent Stirling Falls or the 531-foot Bowen Falls. We were lucky to have our cruise in late August on the first sunny day in three weeks. The rainfall is heavy in this area — up to 275 inches a year, and it is wise to book your bus ride out from Queenstown when it is predicted that the weather will be clear on Milford Sound. If you have time, allow yourself three or four days in Queenstown, so that if one day is stormy you can select another for this adventure.

The luncheon cruises depart at 11 A.M. and at 1 P.M. weather permitting. If you are driving and wish to spend a night at the Hotel Milford on the sound, it is very reasonable, but should be booked well in advance.

Book the day excursion while visiting Queenstown, or if it is part of a bigger tour, make certain you spend two or three days here, so that your chances of seeing this area of great beauty are good.
Write or call:
> Fiordland Travel Ltd.
> P.O. Box 1
> Te Anau, New Zealand

Cost: inexpensive
Fitness rating: easy
Wheelchair access: probable

OR BY AIR

The most costly way to view this natural wonder is to fly over it. Flight-seeing can be arranged. It is a four-hour experience which includes the launch cruise, and allows those who love to fly in small planes a thrilling experience.
Write or call:
> Mount Cook Airline
> 1960 Grand Avenue
> El Segundo, 9th Floor
> Los Angeles, CA 90245
> (800) 468-2665

Cost: moderate
Fitness rating: easy

TASMAN GLACIER ADVENTURE

As we approached the Mount Cook area after leaving Christchurch, New Zealand, our bus driver pointed to the snow-capped mountains and told us, "We also have here some Indian snow — Apache here and Apache there." Our groans delighted him.

Mary Salmon, one of my writing pupils who was with me on this trip, was then a spry grandmother in her 70s with a lively mind and an insatiable curiosity. She wrote, "A visitor to New Zealand is a guest and not just another tourist. New Zealanders like to think that their country is 'God's Country.' They say that after creating the world, He made another country for His own use and enjoyment. He eliminated all deadly creatures. Here, there are no snakes, poisonous insects or wild animals. For added pleasure He put the Islands far away from quarreling areas."

We drew nearer to Mount Cook, the highest mountain in New Zealand at 12,349 feet. The Maoris called it *Aorangi* or Cloud Piercer. Many of the peaks surrounding it are over 10,000 feet. The famous Sir Hilary, who conquered Mt. Everest, practiced on these peaks as a young adolescent.

When older, he stayed at the Hermitage Hotel at the foot of Mt. Cook, and we stayed there years later. It is rustic and in a beautiful setting. The dinners are elegant and in many ways it reminded me of Yosemite's Ahwahnee Hotel. Book this popular hotel well in advance.

In late August we were surrounded by skiers staying at the Hermitage. Many nature hikes are possible from here as well.

As soon as we checked into our rooms we encountered the kea, a common bird here, but unusual to us. It has as much nerve as our blue jay and will eat whatever delicacy you offer it. A dull brownish green, it is more noticeable when it spreads its wings. It is bright red under the wings and it has the hooked beak of the parrot family.

To book the glacier adventure and the hotel —

Write or call:
>The Hermitage Hotel
>Mt. Cook National Park
>South Island, New Zealand
>local phone: 5621-809

Cost: expensive, but no more than a good comparable hotel would be in America. For a splurge it is well worth the price.

Fitness rating: easy

Wheelchair access: Inquire directly. Many rooms are on the ground level. Dining is down several steps.

FLYING OVER THE TASMAN GLACIER

The next morning many in our group took a light plane ride up to the Tasman Glacier. For them it was the high point of our trip. They ascended from 2,500 feet to over 7,000 feet in minutes. Mt. Tasman peaks at 11,470 feet and is the longest glacier in the world if you discount the polar regions. Its length is eighteen miles and its width is two miles. The planes land in the area known as Tasman Saddle at around 7,000 feet.

Although the glacier appeared very near, it was more than a mile away. The passengers were so close they felt as though they could reach out and touch the snow and ice. At one point they thought they saw smoke, but it was an avalanche eight miles away.

When everyone was helped out of the plane, they stood on solid ice more than 600 feet deep. The motors on the plane were never turned off while the group explored the icy glacier, thus preventing any buildup of ice on the wings of the aircraft — a condition which could spell danger.

Write or call:
> Mount Cook Airline
> 1960 Grand Avenue
> El Segundo, 9th Floor
> Los Angeles, CA 90245
> (800) 468-2665

WALKS AND HIKING
IN THE MT. COOK REGION

Advice and maps can be given out by the rangers at Mt. Cook National Park Headquarters, a short stroll from the Hermitage. For longer walks, a guide can be hired through Alpine Guides Ltd. This firm also rents out equipment and they will guide you over the ice and snow, or along the lower paths on beautiful nature trails.

Write:
> Alpine Guides, Ltd.
> P.O. Box 20
> Mount Cook, New Zealand

Cost: moderate
Fitness rating: moderate to strenuous

GLACIER SKIING

Glacier skiing is more costly than hiking. Most avid skiers stay at the Hermitage, take flights up to the glaciers and ski down, sometimes getting in two or three runs a day. The plane has retractable skis on it to facilitate landing. Guides and park rangers fly along with the skiers and stay up there as long as the skiers are there. From the Tasman Saddle, there is a six-mile run downhill through areas of breathtaking beauty and stillness. A guide accompanies you, leading the way and avoiding dangerous crevasses. In 1990, the costs were $275 per person per day. This covered three flights up to Tasman Saddle, lunch, and guides.

This adventure is seasonal, from June to October. For exact current costs for this adventure, or the four day Tasman Treks or half-day heli-hiking adventures —

Write:

> Alpine Guides, Ltd.
> P.O. Box 20
> Mount Cook, New Zealand
> This can also be booked through
> Mt. Cook Airline in Los Angeles.

Cost: expensive
Fitness rating: strenuous

SKIING OUTSIDE QUEENSTOWN

Queenstown is a resort city located on Lake Wakatipu, and it is ideal for vacations. Skiing near here is far less expensive than the glacier skiing.

Coronet Peak is eleven miles out of the city and buses can transport you to the lift area. An all-day lift ticket is reasonable by our standards, as is the rental of skis, poles and boots.

Our group spent five days in this Queenstown area, and that is a good amount of time for Americans with only two weeks of holiday a year, but I would rather explore an area in depth, than visit each city or town for just a few hours. As people grow older, I've observed that they appreciate longer stays in one location. No longer is it a pleasure to pack and unpack each day.

There are many activities here to enjoy, such as a cruise on Lake Wakatipu, and a visit to a sheep farm with an afternoon tea there. Jet boating is for the adventurous. Good dining is everywhere.

If you want an aerial view of Queenstown, walk to Brecon St. and take Skyline Gondola. This will transport you up to 2,400 feet. A good restaurant on the top opens at 10 A.M. The cost of the gondola ride is reasonable. If you have a fear of heights, this is not for you, but if you enjoy magnificent vistas, then treat yourself.

HOME STAYS

From Queenstown you can arrange for delightful home stays, which are offered throughout New Zealand. It is a good way to meet some of the interesting people who live here surrounded by so much natural beauty. Our hostess had recently returned from a six-month holiday — four of those months she had spent exploring India.

Her pavlova, that sweet meringue dessert filled with kiwi fruit and other exotic fruits, was delicious, her lamb dinner superb. Well arranged in advance, while still in California, we were transported to our hosts' farm by a private car and the transfers were included in the price. Their farm overlooked the Shotover River and we watched jet boats whiz by — a popular adventure that originates in Queenstown.

Had our hostess just inherited a great deal of money? Is that how she managed a six-month holiday? No, I have met Australians and New Zealanders all over Europe who are there for several months or a year. Because of their isolation from so much of the world, both the Aussies and the New Zealanders tend to take very long vacations when they travel so far. But they might wait ten years between those very long explorations abroad. They frequently take leaves of absence or pack those long sojourns between job or career changes. Both countries tend to give their employees four weeks off a year with full pay, so they can travel abroad if they wish.

Our host and hostess were both very congenial. He served sherry wine before dinner, and after the dinner, coffee and liqueurs were served in the living room. When we retired for the night — a brisk cool one in late August — our hostess had thoughtfully warmed our beds with the "down under" version of the electric blanket. The heating coils are in the mattress below us instead of in a blanket on top!

Home stays can be arranged through your travel agent or call after your arrival in New Zealand.

Call:

to stay on the South Island —
Farmhouse and Country Home Holidays, Ltd.
Christchurch 427 704
to stay on the North Island —
Farmhouse and Country Home Holidays, Ltd.
Auckland 410 5960

Cost: Costs of a home stay vary enormously. Your price does include your meals, warm hos-pitality, and a chance to make a lasting pen pal.

Fitness rating: easy

Wheelchair access: request this in advance

FARM STAYS

Farm stays are also possible, and you might stay on a sheep ranch, or on one which raises deer. Venison is highly prized as meat in New Zealand, and they raise deer there as we raise cattle. Or perhaps it would be a farm with kiwi orchards. To book a farm stay, you can arrange it here with your travel agent, or —

Write:

to stay on the South Island
Rural Holidays
P. O. Box 2155
Christchurch, New Zealand
to stay on the North Island
Farmstay Ltd. Rotorua
P.O. Box 630
Rotorua, New Zealand

GLOWWORM CAVES

Not far from Queenstown is the small community of Te Anau, and near here another adventure is waiting. Take a 30-minute ride on a boat across Te Anau Lake and you will come to Glowworm Caves. After World War II, these caves were discovered by Europeans and now there are two tours daily — at 2 P.M. and 8 P.M., weather permitting.

If you do visit here, you will be thrilled by the thousand pinpoints of dancing lights. These caves are located in a more remote area than the Glowworm Grotto found deep within Waitomo Caves on North Island.

Call:
> From Queenstown, arrange with local
> Mount Cook Line travel office.

Cost: inexpensive
Fitness rating: easy
Wheelchair access: no

NORTH ISLAND: GOOD ACCESS FOR THE DISABLED

Auckland is the major city on the North Island of New Zealand. If you are disabled and want to explore the city with your spouse or companion, a Dial-a-Ride service offers minibuses which have wheelchair lifts. If possible, book a day or so ahead. Cost is less than for a taxi. The Dial-a-Ride office is located on Erson Avenue in Auckland.

By writing to the New Zealand Tourism Department, 10960 Wilshire Blvd., Suite 1530, Los Angeles,

CA 90024, you may receive a very useful booklet called *New Zealand Access, A Guide for the Less Mobile Traveller.* There is no charge. Published in 1990, it is current and filled with information. Dr. Michael Quigley, an epidemiologist originally by training, has been using a wheelchair for 20 years since he was injured in Vietnam. He now is very active in the world of travel and is editor of *Handicapped Travel Newsletter.*

He wrote the foreword to this useful booklet. After traveling in at least 90 countries to inspect them for wheelchair and handicapped facilities, he now rates New Zealand as one of the best in the world for those who are disabled.

For an in-depth tour of New Zealand, Atlantic and Pacific Tours has a special coach which has features such as a dual-controlled lift and provisions for up to ten wheelchairs. Sixteen additional passengers can be seated comfortably. There are large windows designed so that everyone can see the passing scenery.

Atlantic and Pacific Tours will give you advice on where to stay on the North and South Islands of New Zealand and arrange tours which would be available to you.

Write or call:
> Atlantic and Pacific Tours
> 230 North Mayland
> Suite 308
> Glendale, CA 91206
> (818)240-0538

NORTH ISLAND: HOME OF THE MAORIS

Everyone will enjoy exploring the North Island of New Zealand, as well as the South Island. Auckland itself is home to a third of the population of New Zealand.

It boasts of two harbors, and first time visitors should take a short cruise on *The Pride of Auckland*, a catamaran that holds 80 passengers. This cruise, as is true of the Captain Cook cruise out of Sydney, Australia, gives you a good introduction to the city. You can see the new emerging skyline of Auckland, which has undergone much building in recent years, and the homes built on cliffs on the North Shore.

A good home-cooked dinner with a New Zealand family is a delightful way to spend an evening while in Auckland. The home we visited for a delicious meal was filled with antiques. We were picked up right at our hotels and transported in groups of four to the homes of our hosts in various parts of Auckland.

Outside of Auckland, we passed many kiwi orchards and drove along Waitomo River and then visited the famous caves. Enjoying a subterranean boat trip along an underground river, we were plunged into almost total blackness as we entered the spacious cavern of the Glowworm Grotto. As our eyes became accustomed to the darkness, we saw the tiny lights of millions of the tiny glowworms illuminating the cave above us. It filled us all with a sense of wonder.

In Rotorua where there are big thermal baths, that evening we enjoyed a *hangi*, the Maori version of the Hawaiian luau. The meat had been cooking for hours in a pit filled with steam from the natural thermal activity. The tables were laden with food and one could go back again and again.

We then had two hours of Maori entertainment performed by the Kotuku (which means white heron) group of entertainers. Songs and dances gave the viewers a greater understanding of the Maori culture. We watched dances of love and welcome, and the fearsome *haka* dance, or the dance of war. In the *haka* the male dancers distort their faces, stick out their tongues and flap them about. These weird looking faces are supposed to terrify their enemies.

The next day was spent exploring the model Maori village where we saw the way they must have lived for countless centuries. Continuing on to the thermal area, we gazed in amazement at the geysers gushing up so many feet into the air, boiling mud pools and steaming underground rivers.

Later that same day we visited another area where the awesome forces of nature were manifested. In 1886, Mt. Tarawera erupted and buried the village of the same name in its path. People from all over the world had visited a natural wonder there — a fabled area of silica terraces called Pink and White Terraces. These were destroyed by the molten lava, but now a part of the village ruins have been excavated so that visitors can see how life was led over 100 years ago.

Back in Auckland, a visit to the War Memorial Museum provided a fascinating afternoon spent studying the fine collection of Maori artifacts and carvings.

On the North Island, the traveler meets the Maori people and is able to study their art forms and their history. If one were to compare the North and South Islands, one would say that on the South Island it is the scenery and the great visual beauty which overwhelms the visitor. On the North Island, it is its people — an anthropologist's paradise.

To book this excursion, see your travel agent or —

Write:
ATS Tour Pacific (its New Zealand tours are now offered in conjunction with Horizon Tours, located in New Zealand)
100 North First St.
Burbank, CA 91502

Cost: land cost alone, moderate, but with air included, expensive. A good policy for singles in New Zealand with Horizon Tours is that if you indicate you are willing to share, while on the actual tour in New Zealand, you only need pay the cost of a single. If the tour company does not find someone to share with you, you will have the single room at no extra cost rather than having to pay the single surcharge.

Fitness rating: easy

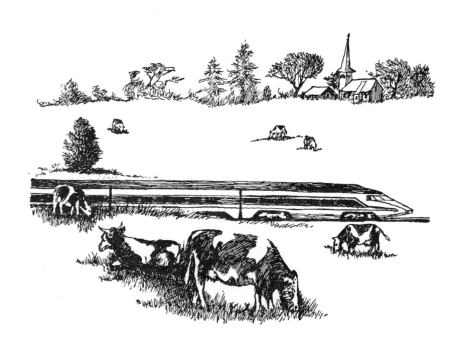

UNUSUAL TRAIN JOURNEYS

VENICE SIMPLON-ORIENT EXPRESS

In 1883, over 100 years ago, the Orient Express electrified travelers by offering unbridled luxury with excellent service. As the train passed through cities with romantic sounding names like Venice and Istanbul, the kings and crown princes of the era began to ride on this fabled train in their own especially appointed cars. It soon attracted the "rich and famous" from all over the world.

The reputation of this extraordinary train grew; and, until World War II, it was a symbol for elegance. After the war, its reputation waned, and by 1978 the train was no longer in service. Its memory lingered as mystery fans encountered this legend through the reading of Agatha Christie's *Murder on the Orient Express* and later the film was made, again heightening interest.

Twenty million dollars was spent to restore the original carriages and engines, and in 1982 the luxurious train began its impeccable service once more.

Now, as you travel on the European continent, your food will be prepared by French chefs and equal to the quality one might expect from a very expensive French restaurant. If you love beautiful clothes and dressing for dinner, this may be the splurge that you would greatly enjoy. One can never be overdressed for dinner on the Venice Simplon-Orient Express. Gentlemen are invited to wear black tie formal wear, but a jacket and a tie will get you in. Women should also wear formal attire, perhaps with a touch of the '20s included. During the day one can dress casually, but I don't think that means jeans or shorts for the ladies.

Your train fare includes all table d'hote meals; but the a la carte menu is extra. Before dinner, one can enjoy a drink in the bar-salon with a pianist playing on a baby grand. Have you ever seen a grand piano on a train?

From February to November this fabled train runs between London and Venice and in the reverse order twice weekly. The trip takes 32 hours and covers over 1,000 miles. Commencing in London, a ferry transports you across the English Channel, but first you are taken to Folkstone aboard a beautifully renovated Pullman car.

At the time of this writing, there were different routings and destinations offered. Service between Venice and London began in late February and the first London to Venice train arrived on February 23 in Venice, that city steeped in history with its many canals, just in time for the famed Venice Carnival.

There are journeys from Vienna to London and from Venice to Vienna via Munich, that Bavarian city of gemutlich charm and culture. One could go to operas in Munich and Vienna and travel in luxury between those two fascinating cities.

There is flexibility in the offerings nowadays because of the tours organized by Venice Simplon. You can stay two nights each in London and Venice, plus a night on the train in the elegant sleeping car. There are also tours which include stays in London and Vienna, a nine-night package offering Venice, Paris and London; London, Venice and Rome; or London, Venice and Florence.

A new routing planned for June 1991 will include Budapest in Hungary as another destination. With departures in each direction every other week, this will be the new itinerary: London-Paris-Innsbruck-Salzburg-Vienna-Budapest; and the return will be: Budapest-Vienna-Salzburg-Munich-Paris-London. To book, see your travel agent or —

Write or call:
>   Venice Simplon-Orient Express
>   One World Trade Center
>   Suite 2565
>   New York, NY 10048
>   (212) 938-6830

Cost: expensive. In 1990 prices: from London to Venice, Vienna or Salzburg $1190 in southbound direction, or $90 less northbound, low season. High season is more costly. For a 'teaser' or just a sampling, one could spend $245 and travel northbound from Venice to Lausanne in Switzerland in the low season from late February through March. It might be enough to see how the 'other half' lives. Costs are considerably higher for the stays in first class or deluxe hotels in addition to the train journey.

Fitness rating: easy

Wheelchair access: yes, but arrange in advance

A JOURNEY BY SEA
ON THE *M.V. ORIENT EXPRESS*

If you want to continue on your journey all the way to Istanbul, that is now possible with a voyage by sea on the *M.V. Orient Express.* Then the romantic names of Piraeus (outside Athens), Kusadasi, Patmos, and Istanbul come alive as you visit these islands and cities you have read about all of your life. These sailings operate between May and

November.

Many Europeans take their cars along because below the lowest passenger decks on this ship is a car ferry. With their cars, Europeans can enjoy the beaches of southern Turkey and drive out from Athens, exploring Greece at their leisure. You can stay for a week or longer at any of the ports of call and then again embark on the ship to sail back to Venice. With a rental car or a car you've purchased in Europe you could get off at one port and then get back on at another port. You need not retrace your steps. Freedom and flexibility present you with many choices, but while on board the *M.V. Orient Express* you are treated to all the pampering of a regular cruise ship.

On this journey by water, you will sail across four seas! After departing every Saturday from Venice, the boat docks in Athens on Mondays, on Tuesdays in Istanbul, Wednesdays in Kusadasi (Ephesus) and later that same day in Patmos. On Thursdays the ship arrives in the afternoon at Katakolon (Olympia) and by Saturday the boat arrives back in Venice.

Therefore, if it's Tuesday it must be Istanbul! The pace of the sailing sounds brisk, but you may elect to take shore excursions which last a few hours, or to get off for a week as I have mentioned.

The cost is not any more than a Caribbean cruise on most cruise lines and less than many, which is surprising. Prices vary according to the type of cabin or stateroom desired and the season of the year you choose to travel. Regular season is May 7 through the first week in July and from mid-September until the end of October. High season is from mid-July to mid-September. Air is an extra cost and shore excursions are optional. To book, call your travel agent to coordinate the flights and other arrangements or —

Write or call:
> Venice Simplon-Orient Express
> New York, NY zip
> (212)938-6830

Cost: low moderate
Fitness rating: easy
Wheelchair access: probable, as with most cruise ships

AUSTRALIAN TRAIN ADVENTURES

One of the advantages of being older is that you generally have more time to spend on your travels because you are either retired or have more vacation time than your younger counterparts.

For a leisurely train journey, you might consider travel on one of the world's great trains, the Indian Pacific, which runs from Sydney to Adelaide to Perth and back.

Whereas the London-to-Venice Orient Express journey lasts 32 hours, the Australian continent is enormous and the journey from east to west lasts twice as long as the European luxury car. It takes 65 hours to travel from Sydney to Perth — a distance of some 2,700 miles. You will travel from the Pacific Ocean to the Indian Ocean and see a great variety in the landscapes as you traverse the continent.

As you leave Sydney, the train crosses the tall and spectacular Blue Mountains. This is an area you should explore when visiting Sydney, because it is only a few hours by car or bus out of this bustling city, and there are organized day trips to the Blue Mountains if you don't wish to go alone. With friends it is an exciting area for hiking and exploring, and well worth taking three or four days to enjoy. This is a photographer's delight with the tall pinnacles of the Three Sisters, the scenic railway which hurtles down a tree-lined gorge and is advertised as the steepest railway in the world, and the brilliant colored lorikeets found here in such profusion. Resort hotels are in this region to welcome you.

But for now, you are off on this train journey, and the train carries you on past the Blue Mountains. You then see the rich pastoral lands of grazing sheep and sleek race horses in New South Wales. As you travel south to Adelaide, you might want to get off and spend a few days, for there is much to see and do in this region.

After climbing aboard again, you pass through wheat fields and see many silos dotting the landscape. West over the Nullarbor Plain, which is a limestone plateau, and then there are 298 miles of straight track — the longest straight stretch of tracks in the world. This might be a good time for forming new friendships or dining on a delicious meal.

Kalgoorlie, that fabled gold town of the last century where fortunes were made and lost, is one of the next towns you may want to explore. Then there are more wheat fields and you reach the coast and the beautiful city of Perth on the Indian Ocean.

You probably would choose our fall months to explore the region around Perth, the capital of Western Australia, because it is famous among nature lovers for its enormous fields of wild flowers, stretching as far as the eye can see. The seasons are reversed from America. If it's our fall, it's spring "down under."

Botanists and horticulturists are unanimous in proclaiming the masses of wild flowers which carpet these valleys and hills around Perth as equal to anywhere in the world for sheer color and beauty.

This is also a popular mecca for Australians in the fall, so you need to book this train for the autumn months well in advance. Most of the cars aboard the Indian Pacific train are first class, but once a week each way a section is added with economical twin accommodations. Request this at time of booking.

Flights across the vast continent of Australia are very costly, so the train already represents a big savings. To give you an idea of its size, Western Australia alone is three and a half times bigger than Texas. In the outback one finds sheep stations as big as all of Tasmania.

On the Indian-Pacific train there is also a piano, and passengers can join in a "sing-along."

As in Europe with the Eurail Pass, visitors from

other countries can purchase an Austrailpass which has a validity for varying lengths of time from fourteen days to three months. This can only be purchased before arrival in Australia, and is not available to Australians. Sleeping accommodations are extra, but are often less than hotel rooms, so you could save money by traveling and sleeping on the train at night, and getting off the next day, refreshed and ready to explore a new destination. You can get off at any station en route, as long as you have made prior arrangements for the stop.

Purchase the pass through your favorite travel agent, or —

Write or call:

> Australian Travel Service/Tour Pacific
> 100 North First Street
> Burbank, CA 91502
> (818) 841-1030

Cost: inexpensive to moderate. The budget Austrailpass is approximately three-fifths the cost of the First Class Austrailpass. They can be purchased for either 14 days or for 90 days.

Fitness rating: easy

Wheelchair access: yes. Notify ATS or your travel agent in advance. Tell them you need wheelchair assistance. Your own might not fit, but could be stored in baggage or folded up. They can provide a smaller, more narrow wheelchair which fits in the train's aisles.

KURANDA SCENIC RAIL

One of my favorite train journeys is a brief one, but if you are in Cairns, Queensland, Australia, it is an extraordinary day spent on a tour called Atherton Tablelands and Kuranda Scenic Rail.

It is a narrow gauge railroad leading through some magnificent country of steep ravines, with lush tree ferns and many tunnels. It must have been quite an engineering feat when it was first built, because much of the terrain looks steep and too rugged for man to conquer.

After one horseshoe turn, fields and gorges carpeted with wild yellow lupin tumbled into view. This area boasts of monsoon rains, and one year 72 inches of rain fell in 72 hours, washing out a portion of the railroad. The men building this track must have faced constant danger.

The very high Barron Waterfall leaves the viewer breathless, and as you arrive at the Kuranda Railway Station you feel you are in the tropics. Hanging ferns, masses of flowers in pots, and staghorn ferns growing out of pieces of bark are everywhere. Air plants or epiphytes are here also, and lovely delicate lavender orchids and wild scarlet poinsettia.

After a snack in the station, by bus you are transported to a restaurant near a swamplike lake. As you board the *Water Duck* you know you are in for another type of adventure. This weird vehicle is at home on land or on the sea. It is an amphibious Army vehicle left over from World War ll and was built by the Americans.

As we glided through a small portion of a rain forest, we saw a strange creature in the water, looking like a tiny dragon. It was an iguana. We saw a paper-like tree — the Scopola — used for medicinal purposes. In drug form it is used to produce twilight sleep, a truth serum, and recently, those "Transderm Scop" patches one places behind the ear to combat motion sickness.

The hanging vines over the water were alive with brilliant blue butterflies and lorikeets, those multicolored parrotlike birds so prevalent in Australia. Golden Slipper vines, lavender bougainvillea, and red blossoms were everywhere.

Of course most of us were screaming with delight every time the *Duck* spanked the water, and two or three of us were quite soaked at the end of the hour's explorations. This expedition was a great favorite with all ages on that day. Two grandmothers were traveling with their teenage grandchildren and the young peoples' delight increased our own.

A good lunch was followed by a bus tour to visit Tinaroo Dam and on to the Orchid House. Then we made a visit to the ancient Curtain Fig Tree with its enormous girth. A group of 20 can be photographed in front if it and the people appear tiny compared to its surface of hanging twisted vines.

On to Lake Eacham, formed long ago in the crater of an old volcano. A beautiful shade of emerald green makes this lake unique. Then on we drove to Lake Barrine, where a few of the hardier souls went swimming. Most of us had tea here — scones and thick cream, and good bracing Australian tea.

Pelicans, a male brush (or scrub) turkey, and many Brolgia, a grey bird in the crane family, were enjoyable to watch.

Traveling down from this lush area through the Atherton Tableland where many crops are raised, we arrived back in Cairns a little after 5 P.M. It had been a wonderful day filled with variety.

This day trip can be booked through your travel agent prior to your arrival if you fly directly into Cairns for your first stop in the South Pacific and know your time in Cairns will be limited, or you can arrange this after your arrival in Cairns. This tour operates daily.

Write or call:
Australian Travel Service/Tour Pacific
100 N. First Street
Burbank, CA 91502
(818) 841-1030

Cost: inexpensive, and a child's fare is available at half the adult's

Fitness rating: easy; suitable for older adults who cannot walk even a block without tiring. This is an adventure which calls only for climbing onto trains and buses and for being eased into the *Water Duck*.

Wheelchair access: no

Flexibility in New Rail Passes Abroad

Most of you are probably aware of the Eurail Pass, which gives the traveler unlimited travel on the railroads of western Europe in seventeen countries. England and Northern Ireland are the exceptions with their own Britrail pass, but even Ireland participates in the Eurail program.

There is now a new offering in Europe which is less expensive than that pass if you wish to stay several days in one location. Called the Eurail Flexipass, it is valid for 21 days and can be used on nine separate days. It is designed for saving you the worry of having to purchase your ticket abroad when your foreign languages may be rusty. It could be very helpful for those who are traveling from one country to another and staying up to a week in one city or area before moving on, particularly if you don't want the hassles of driving in a foreign country. The Eurail Flexipass gives one all the same benefits as the Eurailpass at less cost. It must be purchased in America or Canada before arriving in Europe and can be purchased through any travel agent.

It does not guarantee you a seat unless you make a reservation, but that is relatively easy to do from a phone after arriving in Europe. The first date that you use the Eurailpass is counted as the first date in your 15- or 21-day pass.

For use in all of Europe the savings for a Eurail Flexipass is not great, just the reduction of about an eighth of the price. In 1989 prices, for example, a 21-day Eurail Pass cost $398. A Eurail Flexipass for nine days of travel within a 21-day period cost $340. Children under 12 years pay half fare and under four are free with both plans.

Where savings really occur is in France with its

unique Flexible Railpass. There are two plans available. One is a four-day pass valid for any four days of train travel within a fifteen-day period, and the other is a nine-day pass which is valid for one month.

AN ADVENTURE WITH THE
FRENCH FLEXIBLE RAILPASS

We purchased the four-day pass to be used within the fifteen-day period in 1989, the year of France's bicentennial celebrating its revolution. It was a gala year for France and our group was augmenting the crowds of foreigners who visited France that year to celebrate.

In retrospect we should have chosen another year because of the crowds, but it was festive. With our French Railpasses safely tucked in our pockets, we spent a week enjoying Paris and its environs.

The only day I really felt was too crowded was when we visited Mont St. Michel, that magnificent monastery which is almost cut off from the mainland when the tides are high. Artists have painted this for centuries and Debussy's *Engulfed Cathedral,* or *La Cathedral Engloutie,* was inspired by this historical site, which was an important pilgrimage for Catholics in the Middle Ages. With its unique vistas of sea and sand and tall towers built on top of natural rock promontories, it attracts many to its shores.

Now tourists flock there in droves, climb the hundreds of stairs, explore its ramparts and gaze in wonder at its architecture. Plan, if you can, to visit this on a weekday after the European school children have returned to their classes. I love children, but we visited towards the end of August when most countries have their holidays. That was our error. Since performing Debussy's *La Cathedral Engloutie* as a child myself, I had longed to see Mont Saint Michel, but not with a cast of thousands.

After a week in Paris, we used our French Flexible Pass to travel to Dijon, the capital of Burgundy, where we enjoyed a few days of floating down canals and through locks on an elegant French barge.

Then on to Strasbourg, a city in Alsace which has been tossed back and forth between France and Germany several times in its turbulent history.

After exploring Strasbourg for a few days, we traveled by train back to Paris. The trip was made partially on the TGV, one of the fastest trains in the world. It was an experience in itself to see the countryside whiz by so rapidly. For portions of travel using the TGV, even if one holds the France Flexible Railpass in his hot, sticky hands, one is not guaranteed a seat. A reservation is needed and I called ahead to procure this. The reservation fee was $8 per person, but we were then assured of first class seats.

The big disadvantage of traveling by rail in Europe, even by this relatively painless method of booking, is the shortage of porters. They are almost nonexistent now. Since I was traveling with my mother and other older adults, I found myself running up and down stairs when we had close connecting times — the same sets of stairs several times with each person's suitcases. Sometimes the distance between tracks looks formidable when one has to descend one or two stories of steep stairways, go through connecting tunnels, and climb another couple of stories underground to emerge from the bowels of the earth once more. There should be elevators installed if there are no porters. Then suitcases with wheels would suffice and travelers could manage their own luggage, as in airports. We found only one porter in our four days of exploring France by train — a big drawback.

Travel light is the best advice. Most European train stations in the bigger cities have a storage area for your large suitcases. For a nominal fee you can deposit those monsters for a week or more at a time and travel with a small overnight bag in relative comfort.

There are other financial advantages to the French Flexible Railpass because it gives the bearer a free transfer by rail from Orly or Charles De Gaulle airports to Paris and back. A taxi or a private car can easily cost $60 round trip. You are also entitled to a free one-day Metropass on the Paris subway or the bus system. Other discounts are given on private scenic rail lines and on the entrance fees to several museums.

To book, see your travel agent or —

Write or call:

French National Railroad
360 Post St.
San Francisco, CA 94108
(415)982-1993

Cost: inexpensive; children under 4 years are free

Fitness rating: moderate; strenuous with luggage

Wheelchair access: unknown, but on the TVG wheelchairs could be taken on board if they folded up. The disabled person would need someone ambulatory to help out.

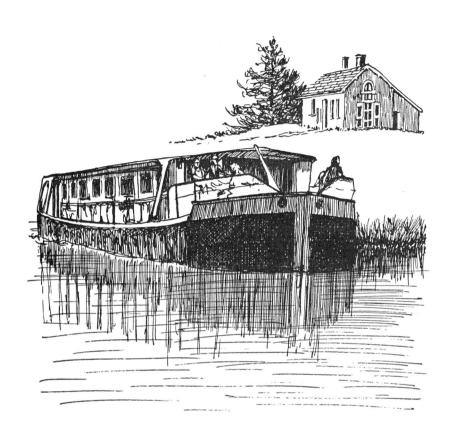

BARGING

ON THE CANALS OF FRANCE

Creme de cassis was our welcoming drink. Later, on another evening, we were to enjoy *Gateau noir avec cassis*, *poulet en la chemise* and *tarte tin-tin*.

Does it all sound like part of a menu for an excellent French restaurant? It should, because aboard our French barge, the *Reine Pedauque*, or the web-footed queen, we feasted at midday and in the evening just as one would in a three-star Michelin restaurant. Curiously enough, however, I don't believe any of us aboard gained weight.

There was healthy exercise available for everyone, even the dog, our mascot. He belonged to Max and Bea, our captain and the chef, who were happily married and living on this luxurious barge.

Our adventure began with a van pick-up in Dijon at the elegant Hotel du Cloche in the heart of the city. We had used our French Flexible Railpass to reach Dijon from Paris. Others had driven to Dijon in rental cars. After a cool glass of *creme de cassis*, a wine drink made with black currants, we were introduced to our week-long companions, and then we were shown to our cabins, where we freshened up a bit.

Afterwards we were all taken into Dijon for a walking tour of the older portions of Dijon in the Antique Quarter. Once the capital of the Dukes of Burgundy, Dijon's history stretches back to Roman times. We made wishes after rubbing the small sculptured owl on the facade of Notre Dame Church and the Milliere House built in the 15th century. Near the Dukes Palace we visited the Tour de Bar built in the 14th century, climbed Gabriel's staircase, constructed in 1733, and thus we became acquainted with each other and with Jean Luc, our guide, and the other navigator aboard the *Reine Pedauque*.

After two hours of exploring on foot, we had all

worked up a fantastic appetite and were driven back to the barge in time for a glass of wine and a brilliant sunset. We were just ten guests, six Americans and four very interesting and charming Australians who had been living in Port Moresby, Papua, New Guinea for several years. One couple, Phil and Cathy Parnell, had lived there for twelve years.

Our dinner one evening was typical of our delicious repasts. It commenced with a half of an avocado filled with smoked salmon, set on red cabbage with herbs and an oil dressing, accompanied by a white wine with a French name I no longer recall. All wines served with the meals were included in the price.

Then came that delightful sounding course, *poulet en la chemise* or chicken in a shirt, which turned out to be a pastry filled with sliced chicken, minced mushrooms, and carrots, with a tomato sauce. The pastry was flaky, buttery and delicious.

With each course a different wine was served, and about six kinds of cheese were served with fruit, including one unusual burgundy-flavored cheese with raisins, somewhat like a French pepper cheese, and a strong tasting goat cheese.

Our dessert was *gateau noir avec cassis*, a white cake with chocolate frosting and black currants with a cream sauce. Coffee was served in the lounge.

The next morning we all started walking between locks and bicycling for an hour or two beside the canal on the tree-lined pathway. By the end of our second evening, we cried, "Help!" and our delightful chef began to adapt some of her recipes and serve us delicious food not quite so laden with rich sauces and cholosterol, although we were later to enjoy frog legs and *escargots* or snails.

The *Reine Pedauque* is the newest hotel-barge in France, yet she has a long history. A paradox? Yes, but a fascinating one. First used 100 years ago as a working barge on the canals of France, which were built in Napoleon's time, the barge was sunk during World War ll so that no German would discover it.

After the war, she was carefully restored and has rich wood paneling throughout. Up to twelve passengers and five crew members can sleep aboard. On the upper deck is a sun deck, a large lounge, a small bar, and a beautiful dining room. On the lower deck are six cabins, all with private baths.

The legend behind the name *La Reine Pedauque* is an intriguing one. One of the Dukes of Burgundy grew tired of his first wife, the Duchess. After somehow getting her sent off to a nunnery, and the first marriage annulled, he installed a new wife in his Ducal Palace. She maliciously spread the rumor that her predecessor had had webbed feet. The tale has been embroidered upon through the centuries, but it is one well known in that region of France.

The crew all spoke both French and English, and as we traveled along the Canal du Centre Saone, we passed through many locks. Our dog would invariably jump off, wag his tail at all the farm animals guarding the locks and then jump in the water for a good swim.

We were in the Burgundy wine region, in a canal near the River Ouche. While floating along the canal, we passed by small villages, exploring some of them on foot. After we left the barge, the group visited a 12th century abbey and a chateau set in a vineyard. The owner introduced his local vintages for his guests at a wine tasting.

The barge was expensive, but this company allowed groups or individuals to stay for only three nights if they wished. This cost roughly half as much as the six-night cruise. The suites had an additional surcharge. It is possible to charter the entire barge for a group of twelve friends if you are very rich or have wealthy friends. The crew stays on board.

For an additional $200 round trip, the company arranges a total spoiling for you if you wish to be picked up by an English-speaking chaffeur at your Paris hotel and taken to the train in style. You are then met in Dijon at the train station.

Other barges operated by the same company with varying prices are *Royal Cognac*, *Le Bateau Ivre* and the *Athos*.

Book through your travel agent, or —

Write or call:
  B and D De Vogue Travel Services
  P.O. Box 1989
  Visalia, CA 93279
  (209)733-7119
Cost: expensive

BALLOONING IN BURGUNDY

The most exciting hour for many aboard *La Reine Pedauque* was a balloon flight over the pastoral fields of Burgundy. Cathy Parnell, our new Australian friend who lives in New Guinea (an island many Americans are afraid to visit), was fearful of this adventure, and had to be persuaded to join in, but five in our group went. They were joined by a portly German gentleman tourist.

We all watched the preparations and I translated for the German tourist into French for the delightful Frenchman who was going to be at the controls. They did not speak each other's language.

Instead of going up in the early morning as many other balloonists do, this was to take place late in the afternoon. The balloon was a kaleidoscope of colors and as it filled with hot air it became immense. The basket was loaded with its human cargo and for one enchanting hour they were airborne. Those of us on the earth watched the balloon lift off until it became a tiny dot on the horizon.

The adventurers returned to the barge about 9 P.M., thrilled and elated. They had watched a glorious sunset as they were coming down. Cathy was very proud of her courage and Bea, our chef, had a light supper for them — at their request — of French onion soup, salads, fruits and cheeses, followed by a *tarte tin-tin* (an upside-down apple tart).

Those of us back on the barge early had enjoyed a French cooking lesson as we watched Bea prepare the delicious tarte, and we had partaken of a heavier dinner of many courses.

In 1989, this ballooning over Burgundy cost more than some of the ballooning in California. The total time spent is close to three hours with all of the preparations before and after, as the balloon is filled with the hot air and later deflated. Champagne was served at the conclusion of the flight. The company's name was Air Escargot, a charming name, but it appeared to be traveling faster than a snail. The ride could be arranged while on board the barge or with your travel agent before leaving the states.

Write or call:
> B and D De Vogue Travel Services
> P.O. Box 1898
> Visalia, CA 93279
> (209) 733-7119

Cost: moderate
Fitness rating: easy
Wheelchair access: no

OTHER BARGE TOURS IN EUROPE

Another company selling barge tours in Europe is called Floating Through Europe. This company handles arrangements for barge trips in Belgium, Holland, the South of France with a tour of Carcassonne's La Cite, a medieval city of ramparts and moats which is fascinating to explore, the Alsace-

Lorraine region of France, and one in the Burgundy wine country, as well.

These are all seven-day, six-night trips and cost approximately the same as those offered by B and D De Vogue Travel. There are no three-day, three- night barging trips offered by Floating Through Europe.

It is possible to rent a "bare" boat barge for exploring the canals of France or England. Then your family and friends are the navigators, the cooks, and the bottle washers. No one is along to spoil you. It is a great family holiday, however, which all ages can enjoy. Those arrangements are handled through other companies. See your travel agent for booking this adventure.

BARGING IN ENGLAND

Floating Through Europe also offers several barging experiences in England. One which sounds very appealing involves floating down the River Avon in a barging adventure called Shakespeare Country. I would recommend this in the late fall after the mobs have departed. Have you ever been to Stratford-upon-Avon in high season? People are walking eight abreast, and it is too crowded to bring one any pleasure.

To reserve, book with your travel agent or —

Write or call:
> Floating Through Europe
> 271 Madison Ave.
> New York, NY 10016
> (212)685-5600

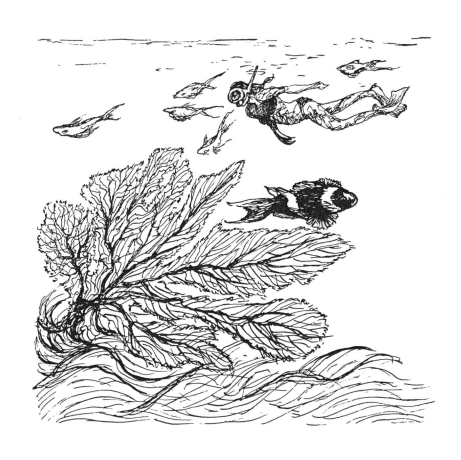

THE GREAT BARRIER REEF

To write of snorkeling and diving and not to mention the Great Barrier Reef would be a mistake. It is one of the most famous areas in the world for its extraordinary coral reefs and for its great variety of tropical fish. Stretching for 1,200 miles from Bundberg to near the coast of New Guinea, it actually comprises two reef systems. More than 1,400 species of fish are to be found here!

I have now visited this reef three times and on each visit I have enjoyed many underwater adventures. There are at least three ways you can experience the Great Barrier Reef and see some of its unique natural wonders.

The first one is my personal favorite. Fly into Cairns, which now often can be your first stop on a flight pattern from America's west coast. One type of ticket allows four stopovers in Australia and New Zealand. After such a long flight, it is wise to unwind and rest for a day in a resort area like Cairns, far from a large bustling city.

HAYLES OUTER REEF
AND GREEN ISLAND CRUISE

For your second day, sign up for the "Hayles Outer Reef and Green Island Cruise." By 9 A.M. in your new time zone you are aboard a big catamaran, spanking along transparent blue-green waters, headed for Green Island. As you look over the sides into the water, you already see some of the fish you will later enjoy in a riotous mass of color and movement.

One of the world's first underwater observatories was created on Green Island in 1954. It still affords the nonswimmer a view of many species of fish. Many red squirrel fish, tiny midnight blue angel fish with bands of bright yellow, the comical clown fish, the iridescent blue and green parrot fish with its lavender and pink markings, the electric blue tang, as brilliant a blue as the Ulysses butterfly, schools of perch, coral trout, and many types of the coral itself in many hues of lavenders, blues, whites, pink and yellow. In all this beauty was a very ugly giant groper — mud-colored with a great natural camouflage.

The resort of Green Island is simple and rustic with basic units, but some day I want to return here and stay on this island for a few nights, snorkeling all day.

On this particular excursion, after a swim in the warm 80° water, we boarded the big "cat" and sailed on to Michaelmas Cay where we had lunch on yet another catamaran moored near the tiny cay.

For over an hour in a glass bottom boat we were guided over the coral reef world, which sometimes appeared only inches below us. Thousands of fish darted about, and we learned about the variety of the coral reef.

Then we went ashore on Michaelmas Cay where we watched hundreds of birds, primarily gannets and sooty terns, and their tiny fledglings in their nesting areas. We did not disturb them and were not permitted to go on to the grass where their nests actually were, but we stood less than six feet from them and could hear them calling out and feel the wind they created as they flew by.

Snorkeling followed for the next hour and a half, opening up new wonders and more species of fish.

All too soon the adventure drew to a close and we caught the cat back to Green Island. People from at least ten nations were in on this special day, and we enjoyed meeting them and becoming acquainted.

This can easily be arranged in Cairns, and departs daily at 8:30 A.M., returning at 5:15 P.M.

Write:

> Hayles Outer Reef and Green Island Cruise
> Hayles Wharf
> Wharf Street
> Cairns, North Queensland, Australia

Cost: inexpensive

Fitness rating: easy, if you don't participate in the swimming

Wheelchair access: unknown, but you could sail as far as Green Island and visit the underwater observatory

QUICKSILVER BARRIER REEF EXPERIENCE

One of the other ways to explore this area is called the *Quicksilver* Barrier Reef Experience. For some reason, this is the one which is always suggested by the tour operators in this country, and I found it a big disappointment. Costing approximately the same amount of money as the previous adventure, it does not offer the variety of experiences nor are any bird sanctuaries visited.

If you depart from Cairns, you are subjected to about ten stops as the bus picks up participants at various hotels and even from campgrounds. An hour and a half is spent just in getting to Port Douglas, but you do pass miles of pristine, deserted beaches.

After you climb aboard the *Quicksilver,* this spacious catamaran transports you out to sea to an anchored platform with an underwater observatory which had a very narrow entryway. From here you could see a few fish. Many people were seasick on the way out to the platform and only about four hearty swimmers dove off the platform to snorkel or scuba dive.

Lunch was served while we were on the platform, turning various shades of green. Because it was a windy day, the water was murky and visibility poor, although those few who snorkeled enjoyed it.

I would suggest signing up for this experience only in the warm months and only if you have good sea legs. This certainly can be booked there in Cairns or in Port Douglas.

Write or call:
    ATS Tour Pacific
    100 North First Street
    Burbank, CA 91502
    (818) 841-1030
Cost: inexpensive
Fitness rating: easy
Wheelchair access: unknown

A DAY SPENT EXPLORING GREEN ISLAND

A far less expensive way to explore this reef is to catch the 8:30 A.M. catamaran out to Green Island with those who are going there to spend a few nights, stay for the day right on Green Island, explore its underwater observatory and then swim and snorkel all day long, using the island as your base. A delicious lunch can be purchased on Green Island. Tropical birds fly overhead and land in the palm trees shielding the tables from the tropical sun, and children laugh and splash and build sand castles nearby.

If you are a nonswimmer, you can still enjoy the underwater observatory, the lunch and the beautiful tropical setting. Snorkeling equipment can be rented right on the island. The same people who were miserable and seasick on the *Quicksilver* spent the very next day delighted and thrilled with this island. I taught my aunt, in her early 70s, and two teenage grandchildren of another friend, also in her 70s, to snorkel. A wonderful intergenerational day.

This is also easy to arrange after arrival in Cairns.

Write or call:
>Hayles Green Island Cruise
>Hayles Wharf
>Wharf Street
>Cairns, North Queensland, Australia

Cost: inexpensive; additional for snorkeling gear rental
Fitness rating: easy to moderate. If you wish to swim for hours, it could be strenuous.
Wheelchair access: unknown, but it probably could be handled.

Tips for Visiting the Great Barrier Reef

The best time to visit the Reef is from the end of April through all of October, although our first trip there was in February and it was enjoyable. Weather then, however, is unpredictable, and this area is subject to very heavy monsoon-like rains. In the summer months there is an invasion of sea wasps or box jellyfish. Their sting can be fatal, so the miles of deserted beaches in Queensland are no accident. Warning signs are posted during those months. There are no jellyfish out at Green Island or at the many other islands. The jellyfish are in close to the shore of the mainland.

You will read of the many romantic islands between Townsville and Cairns bearing exotic names such as Orpheus Island, Magnetic Island, Lizard Island, Dunk Island, but these are, for the most part, elegant resorts set on tiny islands which are not in the Barrier Reef. Some are wonderful for the naturalist to explore because they feature rain forests. Others, like Lizard Island, are known to sports fishermen who have wealth and wish to catch marlin. Only Green Island and Heron Island, which is reputed to offer the best scuba diving, are actually on the reef.

SAILING IN THE WHITSUNDAYS

Many of the islands I have mentioned belong to the Whitsunday Islands. Captain Cook named the area the Whitsunday Passage in 1770 when he sailed past some of these islands on the feast of Whitsunday, or Pentecost.

(Captain Cook on another occasion gave the kangaroo its name while exploring a different area of Australia. He had watched these giant marsupials hopping about and asked a native Aborigine, "What is it called?"

The native replied, "Kangaroo."

Captain Cook promptly called the strange creature *kangaroo*, not realizing that in the Aborigine language, it meant, "I don't know.")

The Whitsunday Islands were not much more appropriately named, but they would be delightful to explore with a sailboat or on a yacht.

For as little as $390 per person (at this writing) you can arrange for seven nights of sailing aboard a sixteen-and-a-half-meter ketch, the *Cygnus.* It comes with a skipper, and camping equipment is on board. You camp out at night on deserted beaches on islands which are not inhabited.

There is a larger sailboat, the *Golden Plover,* which is a 33-meter brigantine with many tall sails. It looks like a historic sailing ship with its big square sail and its fore-and-aft mainsail. It is the oldest Australian-built sailing vessel. On board are camping equipment and a crew which even includes a dive master to work with certified divers.

Both of these sailing adventures are offered by Coral Sea Lines. To request information —
Write or call:
> ATS Tour Pacific
> 100 North First Street
> Burbank, CA 91502
> (818) 841-1030

Cost: inexpensive
Fitness rating: moderate
Wheelchair access: no

RENT-A-YACHT

Does a yacht sound far out of reach financially? It need not be, if you wish to rent one for a few days in this region of the world.

Every Monday during the months of good weather conditions, you can venture forth on a yacht, complete with a skipper on board. Called the Whitsunday Sailing Adventure, this company arranges five nights and six days of sailing where you take an active role aboard their yacht. If you share twin accommodations, your cost can be quite low. You are invited to help prepare meals with the cook in the galley and help the skipper with the sails on deck.

The guests fish if they wish, and frequently one of the nights is spent on one of the islands, feasting and dancing at one of the resorts. When my husband and I stayed on Dunk Island for a few days exploring the rainforest, we met some of these island-hopping visitors who came ashore to dine and dance and swim. By midnight they were back on board their own sailboat or rented yacht.

If they came ashore in the late afternoon they would find many attentive fathers clustered around the swimming pool. I have never seen so many men willing to babysit and watch their small children learning to swim. It might have been because many of the women staying here were swimming in topless bathing suits!

If you wish to rent a yacht and be your own skipper, the minimum number of nights is seven. You have to demonstrate your ability before sailing off, and if you only sail on weekends as a hobby, a knowledgeable sailor will come on board and spend a couple of hours briefing you. Radios, linens, and a complete galley are on board.

For information, contact your travel agent, or —

Write or call:
> Bernie's Whitsunday Rent-A-Yacht
> Shute Harbor, Queensland PMB 25 MacKay
> Queensland, Australia 4741

Cost: varies widely, according to size, from moderate for a Holland 25-foot sailing yacht to expensive for a 47-foot Woodward sailing yacht.

For a motorboat, a 30-foot cruiser is moderate, a 35-foot motor cruiser is expensive. A security bond of $500 (at this writing) is required before setting off on this adventure, and is refunded after the vessel is inspected upon your return. Or you may purchase for $100 a damage waiver form of insurance, valid for seven days, and then the $500 is instantly refunded.

Fitness rating: moderate to strenuous

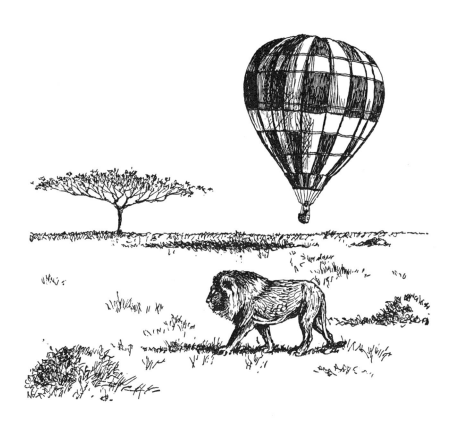

OF OSTRICHES AND ELEPHANTS

ADVENTURES IN SOUTH AFRICA

I realize that nowadays not many Americans visit South Africa, but ten years ago it was a more popular destination. I had read Alan Paton's *Cry, the Beloved Country* and been profoundly moved by this poignant story, but it also made me long to see this country he described.

It is indeed a country of great physical beauty and even in 1980 we saw evidence of many changes — changes that were not mentioned in our newspaper coverages. For the most part, our group stayed in Holiday Inns and they appeared to be fully integrated. Many black guests were staying at each of the hotels we visited, and in one resort town called Wilderness, located right on the Indian Ocean, the Holiday Inn seemed to have guests in equal proportions of Indians, blacks, and whites. We all stood in one buffet line for our delicious meals and I saw no difference in the type of service offered.

For viewing wildlife and visiting some of the great natural wonders of the world, I would recommend touring South Africa as soon as our government lifts its sanctions. The government there is now attempting to make many changes, and as the blacks residing there gain more rights and privileges, it will help their economic status if tourist dollars once more add to their nation's wealth.

The chapter on our treatment of the American Indians is as controversial as South Africa's treatment of the blacks. As a world traveler, I like to visit a country and form my own opinions. Mark Twain once wrote, "Travel is fatal to prejudice, bigotry, and narrow-mindedness."

EXPLORING CAPE TOWN AND ITS ENVIRONS
Cape Town is called one of the most beautiful cities in the world. Historically it is fascinating, for its history stretches back to the 1600s. While in

Cape Town, ride the cable car high up above the city to the peak of Table Mountain. From this vantage point you have magnificent views of Cape Town and you also see the shores of the Atlantic Ocean far below. On the ledges nearby were little *dassies*. A dassie is a strange creature about the size of a cocker spaniel puppy. It is also called a rock rabbit and likes to accept bits of food from your hand.

Driving out from Cape Town we came to Stellenbosch, a carefully preserved town which is nearly 300 years old. Many of the roofs are thatched, and there was a profusion of flowers. Ranunculi were in full bloom. The big town square was bordered with stately oaks. We watched a weaver bird weaving a nest. The female begins to build the strangely shaped nest, which is almost persimmon-shaped, but much larger — at least the size of a coconut. The male then flies in, and if not satisfied, he improves upon it.

Stellenbosch is a small university town, a bit like Oxford. Much of Stellenbosch has spread out around the college. The Afrikaans University is here and the classes are taught here in Afrikaans. At the university in Cape Town the teaching is in English. All races go to all of the universities in South Africa.

Eating lunch in the restaurant on the premises of Stellenbosch Winery was a gastronomic treat. We were given a room for our small group. High up on the white walls was a dark wooden ledge lined with old dishes of delft blue. Old chests with brass fittings and other furniture looked as though the pieces had traveled from Holland with the early settlers long ago. Food was delicious everywhere we ate in South Africa. On this occasion we were served wine, soup, homemade dark bread, unsalted sweet butter, cooked pumpkin with brown sugar, pot roast and mushrooms and a rich bread pudding with raisins — a far cry from my half of a sandwich at home in California.

The next morning we drove out to the Cape of Good Hope, which was extraordinarily wild, and the area evoked an earlier time in history. We passed baboons and ostriches, free and in their native habitat. A funny little bus met us and took us up the steep drive to an outlook. From here we gazed down at the sharp treacherous cliffs where more than 70 ships crashed and sank to the bottom of the sea in earlier days.

It is here that the Indian and Atlantic Oceans meet and we could almost see the differences in the currents below. We were told that there is nearly a 15° difference in the temperatures of the two oceans. The Indian Ocean is warmer and more tropical.

I had organized a botanical tour for the college and had invited Dr. John Thomas, a botany professor from Stanford University, to accompany us. His knowledge greatly enhanced our enjoyment.

With him we visited Kirstenbosch Botanical Gardens, located on the Southeastern slopes of Table Mountain in Cape Town. All of the plants here are indigenous to South Africa and the great variety of protea is quite remarkable. Protea is named for Proteus, a god found in Greek mythology who was able to assume many forms. From our botany professor we learned many of the Latin names, but today I remember that we saw nearly 40 species of those we common mortals call "pincushions." Long tentacles spreading out from the centers make these seem related to some underwater sea creatures like the sea urchin with sharp spines. The best months to visit Kirstenbosch are from August to October, when the spring flowers bloom.

The enormous pink protea cynaroides is perhaps the only Latin name I can still recall. It has an enormous blossom and somewhat resembles the blossom on an artichoke plant. But I do remember acres of colorful protea here and in the wild in the cape area. If you are an avid student of botany, this area of the world offers many species which are only found in the wild here, although attempts to cultivate them elsewhere are quite successful.

A TOUR OF AN OSTRICH FARM; EXPLORING THE CANGO CAVES

This strange beast, the ostrich, looks like it is part turkey and part giraffe. It will drink water but can live for months without drinking any at all. One of its nicknames is *camel bird.*

The easiest way to get to the area of the ostrich farms in South Africa is to fly from Cape Town into Oudtshoorn Airport, which is tiny and charming, with an old world quality. Flowers were planted all around the outskirts of the runway and these blooms reminded me of the Irish and English train stations.

After landing here and climbing out of our small, 44-passenger plane, we were first taken to the Cango Caves. This is usually included in the same day's excursion as to the ostrich farm, because both attractions are in the same region.

The Cango Caves are of limestone and are formed in interesting hues of greens and occasionally pink. One set of formations is called the organ pipes, and sometimes concerts or sound and light productions are given down here in a natural stagelike setting.

The Cango Caves were made a national historical monument in 1938, and at least 80 caverns are now open to the public. Long ago the bushmen knew of their existence, and then in 1780 the caves were rediscovered. *King Solomon's Mines* was written after Rider Haggard visited these unique underground chambers. They rival our Carlsbad Caverns in size and grandeur.

Not more than a half hour's drive from the caves, we came to Highgate Ostrich Farm. We learned much about the ostrich on that day, and now that a few American farmers are beginning to develop ostrich farms here, I would hope that one or two of them would open their ranches to the public eventually as their stock multiplies. Ostriches are fascinating creatures and both the American public and the farmer should profit from the visits.

We were told that the male ostrich mates for life. If his female dies he never takes another, but if he dies, she will mate again. They have been known to live for 85 years, and one female on an ostrich farm was still laying eggs at the age of 72. The male builds the nest, but if the female doesn't like it, he must build it over and over again. One male has had to make fourteen nests and his lady love is still not happy. Does this sound like some human behavior?

At Highgate Ostrich farm we were able to sit on an ostrich if we wished. Mine felt very soft and downy and loved to be scratched behind her ears or have the back of her neck massaged. My roommate was a good horsewoman, and rode an ostrich longer than anyone in our group. There was an ostrich race with several jockeys at a small race track.

At Highgate we saw tiny baby ostriches and many females sitting on the gigantic nests. For lunch we had an ostrich omelette. One egg equals 24 chicken eggs, but it's rather strong in flavor, so milk is added. It makes an enormous meal — the equivalent of 32 chicken eggs, counting the nutritional value of the milk!

Dried ostrich meat resembles beef jerky. Ostrich meat is cholesterol-free and American farmers beginning to work with ostriches hope to sell the meat within a few years. The hides make good leather products.

Right now, here in the states, the cost to the

ostrich farmer for purchasing stock is staggering —
$2,000 for a chick, $25,000 to $35,000 for breeding
adults!

Write:

> Hoopers Highgate Ostrich Show Farm
> Posbus/P.O. Box 94
> Oudtshoorn 6620
> South Africa

Cost: inexpensive. The cost is minimal for a visit to the
ostrich farms and the Cango Caves once you are in the
area. The expense is in getting there! (In 1980, the tour
to the ostrich farm was under $2.00!)

Fitness rating: moderate to strenuous; many steps in
the caves. Easy for the ostrich farm.

Wheelchair access: not for the caves, possible for the
ostrich farm

HIDING IN A BLIND;
VISITING A PRIVATE GAME RESERVE

Have you ever had to compete with wart hogs and
baboons while landing a small plane? Our view out
of the small 32-passenger plane as we circled
Skukuza Airport in the Eastern Transvaal was of
dozens of those comical wart hogs rushing about,
their small tails straight up in the air like so many
little flags.

Soon we were in Kruger National Park, driving
through part of it to reach the private game reserve
of Landolozi. En route we saw many giraffes, zebras,
impalas, and camera-shy baboons. After morning
tea in a rustic lodge which had excellent viewing
areas, we were driven to a small lake where dozens

of big glistening humps were actually hippos submerged in water.

After a delicious lunch, three of us were taken to a blind where we spent about three hours. The others rested, but we had many sightings from our vantage point. Armed with an ice chest of soft drinks and beers, we were up high in a small hut on a raised platform overlooking a pond.

Stately giraffes sauntered by. Zebras came to drink, as did the kudu and many tropical birds. Then, while the other two were resting, I had my biggest thrill. A leopard slunk down to the pond, first looking warily to her right and to her left. She was a beautiful creature. I told my roommate, Maureen, and together we spotted the mate hiding behind a tree.

After we were picked up, our guide became very excited. No one had seen a leopard for a month or two on this land. Our tracker discovered that two tiny cubs had been hiding in the bush as well, and our driver spent the next hour and a half driving wildly around in the land rover trying to find the leopard family again, but there was not a glimpse.

Then we saw a rare white rhino, and after dark a tiny marmoset up in a tree. Everywhere there were herds of impala, and we saw several steenbok and the nyala, an antelope-like creature.

Our dinner that night was around a huge campfire in a great circle made up of tables and benches. There were 21 guests in all. Our rondavel, a small round hut, had one bedroom with a modern bath. A shower felt good, and after a short night we arose before dawn to go game viewing. Many different animals were seen on this drive.

All too soon, we had to catch another plane and return to civilization. When going to a game reserve, allow yourself enough time to savor the experience. Stay two or three nights in each area.

Book with your travel agent, or —

Write:
> Londolozi Game Reserve
> 26 Stanley Ave.
> Auckland Park
> 2092 Johannesburg, South Africa

Cost: moderate
Fitness rating: easy

KRUGER NATIONAL PARK;
VISITING A PUBLIC GAME PARK

When I later spent two days in Kruger National Park, I was disappointed. If you have the discretionary extra funds, try to stay at a private game park like Landolozi. It is disconcerting to view wild animals in a bus, even though our bus was small and held only 20 people. We were not allowed to leave the paved roads, which is probably excellent for the ecological environment and for the wild creatures, but we were often too far away for photography.

This would be an excellent place for game viewing if you are in your 80s or suffer from arthritis and like a smooth ride at all times. In Kenya and on private game reserves, the vehicles take off over some rough terrain, but the photographing opportunities are endless. You must decide which is best for you.

Kruger National Park is rightfully one of the most famous game sanctuaries in the world. It has 7,700 square miles and is criss-crossed by 1,500 miles of roads. If you rented a car you could probably go down all the little side roads and see far more than we did. In addition to herds of giraffes, zebras, baboons, and impalas, there is the strange looking blue wildebeast and over 1,200 lions. Elephants are in the more northern portion of the park. Less frequently seen are the eland, the roan antelope, leopards, cheetahs and the tiny nocturnal cats.

Go in the summer if you are an avid birdwatcher. Go in the winter to view the big game because the grass is closer to the ground and the animals are more visible as they seek out the water holes.

Some of the creatures we spotted on our early morning drive before breakfast were a family of baboons, a grey dakir, at least twelve giraffes, two sable antelopes looking regal and magnificent, yellow billed hornbills, wildebeast, and a pride of lions.

Later, we saw many storks, kudus, vervet monkeys with little white faces, several hippos, a grey kite eagle, many Egyptian geese, a crocodile, and several elephants crossing the road in front of us. We were asked not to move or make loud noises — the elephants could have shaken up our small bus!

After a delicious lunch at Sabie-Sabie, we saw Burchell zebras, more elephants, whimsical wart hogs, and about six zebras grazing with at least 20 impalas.

Kruger has excellent overnight accommodations in rondavels and cottages at eleven different rest stops. The restaurants serve good, hearty fare. It is a thrill to step out of your rondavel in the evening and hear the night creatures prowling and the various bird sounds. Guards are near at hand to protect visitors. Because these rest stops are far apart from one another you don't have the experience of seeing wall-to-wall tents and trailers as in Yosemite National Park.

Reservations may be made a year in advance. To reserve, see your travel agent, or —

Write:
> The National Parks Board
> P.O. Box 787
> 0001 Pretoria, South Africa

Cost: inexpensive

Fitness rating: easy

Wheelchair access: probable with a privately rented auto since this is a national park

A TOUR OF KENYA: HUNTING FOR WILD CREATURES WITH A CAMERA

For an adventure that you will never forget, at least once in your lifetime you should splurge and travel to Kenya for a photo safari.

You might never wish to visit a zoo again. After

photographing creatures in the wild and viewing them on game drives early in the morning and in the late afternoon in such exotic sounding parks as the Masai Mara, the Amboseli National Park, or Tsavo West, it is difficult to get excited about a poor animal locked behind bars in a city zoo.

The film *Out of Africa*, with its beautiful photography of the wild animals and the tragic love story it depicted, caused many Americans to have a wish — that they too would someday see the magnificent beasts in their native habitat.

I escorted a group there in 1987 and our adventures began before we even left the Los Angeles Airport. We were bumped up to business class on our KLM flight by six prize-winning race horses, two elegant cars, and a trainer!

The entire back section of tourist class was blocked off for these high kicking spirited beasts, and we were contentedly ensconced in business class where we were spoiled.

Later we talked to a few unhappy smokers in another group who remained near the partition. They were not so delighted with their horsey neighbors, claiming that they could hear them kicking in the night and could detect a barnyard aroma.

Our flight was direct and nonstop from Los Angeles to Amsterdam. After an afternoon of sleeping and showering in Amsterdam, we flew on to Nairobi. It is a very long flight to Africa and if you wish to enjoy your trip, try to arrange a stopover each way in Europe en route.

Arriving in Nairobi the next morning, we were met and taken to the historic Norfolk Hotel by our guide, Joseph. A very knowledgeable black Kikuyo, he was proficient in four languages: French, English, Swahili and the language of his Kikuyu tribe which comprises 80% of the population in Kenya.

That afternoon I had arranged for us to visit Karen Blixen's (Isak Dinesen's) home where *Out of Africa* was filmed. We visited her estate and saw her study, where much of her writing took place. The grounds were well kept and spacious. Later we were driven to the final resting place of Denys Finch-Hatton.

Back to the Norfolk Hotel with its extensive gardens and tall aviaries of colorful African birds, where most of us dined early and retired by 9 or 10 P.M., local time. (I've found that it is easiest to combat jet lag by forcing myself to stay up if possible and then to retire at night in the new time zone. If you retire upon arrival, you may be up at 2 A.M. in an unknown hotel in a foreign country, unable to enjoy any activity until the next morning.)

Early the next day we left Nairobi in our Nissan Datsun vans, each one limited to six people so that everyone had a viewing seat. The vans had been modified in Kenya so that they had raised open air roofs. We could stand and take photos without glass to distort the picture whenever the van was stopped.

When we saw our first stately giraffe a couple of

hours out of Nairobi, we were awestruck. At first it looked unreal, like a statue, but as we watched it move elegantly forward, we realized we had just seen our first wild creature, unhampered by bars, free to roam wherever it pleased.

The national parks of Kenya offer many different types of wild animal viewing. Although technically you could arrange to stay full time in one park and in one lodge, you would miss the immense variety of landscape and wild life that makes Kenya such an exciting destination.

Portions of Kenya resemble California. Tsavo West National Park is vast and boasts of more than 8000 square miles. It is noted for its birdlife, and we saw many species. Even on our first morning rest stop, we watched golden palm weavers working on their nests. These birds often weave apartment-style nests where 30 or 40 bird families all live together, so the nests hang in great clusters. As we drove on towards our game lodge we spotted zebras, more giraffes and herds of wild gazelles and baboons.

Our first lunch in the bush held surprises. My roommate and I sat near the edge of the open air dining area of the Kilaguni Lodge to watch the storks and baboons. Twice a baboon snatched a portion of my roommate's lunch. He thrust his paw into her plate and gobbled down a fistful of food. Before she went through the buffet line again, we moved further away. Since it was a sumptuous hot buffet she said she brought back a better selection each time!

At breakfast the next morning a mama vervet monkey, her baby clinging to her, leapt down, snatched a man's breakfast roll from his dish and scampered up on to a rafter, where she defiantly chomped on the roll.

On this safari, the eating was prodigious. If there was an early morning game drive, we would sip hot tea or coffee and have biscuits before dawn. Returning at 9 or 9:30 a.m. we would have enormous buffet breakfasts featuring about 30 selections.

A lecture might follow, or we would drive to a new area, or a new park, where a different type of animal might be viewed. Another enormous buffet would be awaiting us for lunch at about 1:00 or 1:30 p.m. One elegant luncheon repast had an entire table groaning with about 20 tempting desserts, in addition to the usual buffet selections. Our dinners were always served to us at about 7:30 or 8 p.m., and they were leisurely and unhurried.

At Samburu Lodge after a delicious dinner we were seated around our table, sipping coffee and enjoying dessert, when we heard a very loud purring overhead. Glancing up, over the door jamb on a high ledge was the biggest house cat I'd ever seen.

Buff colored with black spots, it had leopard markings, was slender and had wide large ears. Some two feet and a half in length, its tail was half as long as its body. Not a household cat at all, but a serval (felis leptailurus serval). She was a new creature to most of us, and hungrily ate a bowl of food the help put on the ledge for her, her eyes shining fiercely in the dimly lit room. The next day we saw her again, with her brood of kittens.

Our second night was spent at Kilaguni Lodge in Tsavo National Park, which covers 8,000 square miles. We had by then seen so many storks, baboons and elephants that we were almost overwhelmed. While dining that night we watched a herd of elephants approach a well lit watering hole. In silence we watched a drama unfold. A baby elephant tumbled in the water and cried out plaintively. Immediately the herd gathered protectively around in a circle so that no natural enemy could destroy the baby, and two adults patiently rescued the infant with their trunks and then guided him firmly along.

At a later date, at Amboseli Serena Lodge, I traipsed back and forth several times between our room, the farthest out, and the main lodge, stopping frequently to visit one of my friends who was fighting "tourista." Near the entrance to the lodge I was startled to see two well armed Masais, with guns and tall spears, standing motionless.

About ten minutes after my last trek back to our room, the shout went out. "Lion! Lion!" Racing by our door with a pounding of feet, those guards chased the lion out into the night. The beast had come down my own path and I had just missed a very close encounter.

TWO WORLD-FAMOUS PLACES
TO STAY IN KENYA:
MOUNT KENYA SAFARI CLUB
AND TREETOPS

Two of the most exciting places where we stayed deserve to be singled out. On our ten-day safari we stayed one night each at the Mount Kenya Safari Club and at Treetops. Both are world-famous.

The Mount Kenya Safari Club was founded by William Holden and it is truly luxurious if you are lucky enough to be placed in one of the villas. The rooms in the lodge itself were going to be renovated because they seemed ordinary and needed refurbishing. I was fortunate and was placed out in a villa. Our bedroom was off an enormous sitting room where there were three big sofas, a huge fireplace, and a complete bar plus big viewing windows. Original paintings and a magnificent rug were hung on the white walls.

With the beamed wooden ceilings and hardwood floors, I felt as though I were the guest in a wealthy private home. Best of all, I could just step outside in the early dawn to stand near our own private pond where a lone heron was already fishing. The ugly mariboo storks awoke in the trees and soon vied with each other for the best fishing spot, fending one another off with their bills.

The dinner the night before had been an elegant one. It was our only night where men were required to wear a jacket and tie to dinner. We glimpsed some of the rich and the famous dining.

Later, after breakfast the next day we visited the area on these 100 private acres where rare and endangered species are kept. Stephanie Powers, the star of the TV series *Hart to Hart,* is the chairwoman of the William Holden Wildlife Foundation, and she came over and talked with Mother and gave her an autograph. It was here that we saw the extremely rare bongo, a creature about the size of an elk. It is a deep chocolate brown with white stripes.

You can also stand in front of the Mt. Kenya Safari Club with one foot on each side of the equator. With Mt. Kenya towering over the entire landscape, it has a powerful effect upon its guests. Everyone of my group wishes to return and stay here two or three nights.

Treetops was very different. Treetops is a three-story lodge supported by 40-foot stilts. We overlooked a salt lick and a watering hole which attracted many animals. Whereas the Mt. Kenya Safari Club is elegant, modern and blessed with all the amenities, Treetops is rustic, historic, and offers only basic simple rooms with shared bathrooms down the hall. The Club has original paintings on its walls, and Treetops has photographs of all the famous people who have visited here, including Queen Elizabeth. She was staying at Treetops on the day that her father died suddenly, making her the queen. For such visitors, there are suites with private facilities.

We took only an overnight bag to Treetops and left everything else at the Outspan Hotel ten miles away.

Here the humans were in the big giant cage and the wild creatures were free to roam where they wished. Once we were inside the lodge, we were not allowed to leave. Tea was served up on the top deck open to the heavens, and we then found good viewing areas behind glass or down in an area designed like a blind. We could see out, but the creatures couldn't see us.

We first saw small timid creatures, the tiny duiker, impala, and the colobus monkey. Then the cape buffalo appeared in large numbers, darkening the horizon with their approach. They are vicious and if they attack a living creature, including man, they will fight to the death. All the other animals vanished, fearing for their lives. The elephants came in untold numbers towards dusk.

Our exciting afternoon was followed by a delicious dinner. My roommate and I climbed up to the top deck and stared at the stars for a long while. It was the clearest viewing we had of them, for there was no artificial lighting around. We had hoped to be awakened that night if the guard saw a leopard, for then the guests receive a discreet knock on their doors, but there were to be no unusual nocturnal visitors that night. Awakening before dawn, I sneaked out of our room, and watched the sky light up with many colors as dawn arrived. Another unforgettable day had begun.

MASAI MARA NATIONAL PARK

A few days later found us in the Masai Mara National Park, where all of the big game can be found. It is located southwest of Nairobi and totals 692 square miles. Here we saw chettahs, hundreds of elephants, giraffes, zebras, wildebeest, and cape buffalo. The delight here is in driving up close to a pride of lions and watching the mother wash her cubs. She lets them nurse, letting out a yawn at the sight of yet another vehicle. For eighteen or more years people have driven up and taken pictures of these tawny great beasts. The lions now ignore the cars and vans. But man should never get out of his car in their presence. Anyone walking towards them would probably be attacked.

Almost everyone in my group would love to return to Kenya some day. The warmth of her people and the hospitality makes one long to return. It is a suitable adventure for anyone at any age who enjoys good health. Two people with me were in their 80s and another woman, traveling with her daughter, celebrated her 89th birthday in our expanded group of adventurers. She participated in every activity.

The only possible drawback might be that the roads in Kenya are not good. On game viewing drives, the vehicles leave paved roads behind, and the ride can be bone shaking and dusty, but exhilarating. Around every curve is a thrill!

If you do not wish to be shaken up by such conditions, there are flying safaris which are more expensive, but may be worth it. Fly into each game reserve and view the animals from van windows.

To book any of these Kenya adventures, call your favorite travel agent or —

Write or call:
> KLR International Inc.
> 1560 Broadway,
> New York, N.Y. 10036
> (212)-869-2850

Cost: expensive
Fitness rating: easy
Wheelchair access: no

BALLOONING IN KENYA

For an additional fee of between $250 and $300 (at this writing), you can decide on your last day in the Masai Mara National Park to arise early and go on a hot air balloon safari.

With the Serengeti below and the gentle giraffes and elephants in great numbers visible in the early morning light, the balloons seem to undulate as they rise into the air and then dip towards the tree tops. Termite mounds protrude from the ground like stalagmites. Lions, wart hogs and other wild creatures are visible below, grazing and awakening also to a new day.

Dr. Grace Devnich, M.D., took such an ascent by balloon not long ago, while in her late 70s. She wrote, "Thompson gazelles leaped, impalas exploded beneath us, while zebra dazzled with their stripes. Cape buffalo and wildebeests dotted the plains amid rare acacia thorn trees."

After an exhilarating hour high in the air, the balloon brought them back to earth and to reality.

She describes the conclusion to her adventure with the following words.

"Men laid propane tanks around an outstretched canvas, just off the ground, padded them for seats, set out spears around the area — for protection of course — and soon a table was set. Champagne was uncorked with great pops, but before the first sip, we raised our glasses in cheers for this once in a lifetime, thrilling, 'swinging' experience."

To book this it is wisest to arrange it in advance with your travel agent or the tour company and prepay. Some wanted to go, but could not, after arriving at the Masai Mara because the balloon rides were fully booked.

Write or call:
> KLR International Inc.
> 1560 Broadway
> New York, NY 10036
> (212) 869-2850

Cost: expensive
Fitness rating: easy

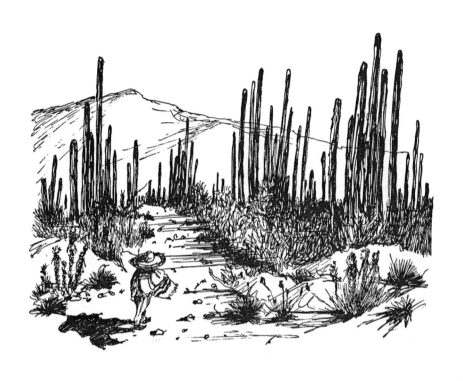

BAJA CALIFORNIA ADVENTURES

A WHALE OF AN OUTDOOR EXPERIENCE
Sven Olof Lindblad's Special Expeditions has been offering fascinating seafaring adventures for years now. Following in the footsteps of his famous father, who offered unusual journeys all over the world, Sven Olof has carved out an important niche for himself with beautifully appointed ships which take

the discriminating passenger to unusual ports of call and on nature viewing expeditions.

The ships, *M.V. Sea Lion* and *M.V. Sea Bird*, each hold a maximum of 70 passengers. Everyone enjoys an outside cabin, a real plus. Because the ships have a shallow draft they can be maneuvered into waters where bigger vessels might run aground. All cabins have private baths and windows or portholes. You can tell whether it is night or day! There is one seating for meals — everyone can be served at the same time. A physician is on board, and naturalists will give passengers the advantage of their knowledge.

The peak time of the migration of the California gray whales is in January and February of each year. The fourteen-day itinerary is offered during those two months each year. Baja California has been called "Mexico's Galapagos," as it has an incredible variety in its sea life and animals on shores.

In addition to the gray whales you may see other members of the whale family — humpbacks like San Francisco Bay's errant Humphrey, finbacks, blues and orcas. Dolphins also are abundant here. Sea lions cavort with you while you snorkel and you see a teeming underwater world of tropical fish. Overhead fly magnificent frigatebirds, blue-footed boobies, brown pelicans, and other, smaller birds.

On this adventure, you will fly from Los Angeles to Loreto, where you will spend one night visiting a mission and exploring the former capital of California, long before it was divided by the boundaries we have today.

You will drive to San Carlos, where you will board the ship, and for the next three days you will be in Bahia Magdalena, a deep bay and the birthplace of most of the thousands of gray whales which migrate here each year from the Arctic. Spending three days near the lagoons where the calving will be a thrilling experience — one you will never forget. By Zodiac inflatable boats, passengers can come in very close to these giants of the sea which were once almost hunted to extinction.

You'll see not only the whale nursery but the breeding grounds for frigatebirds and many other shorebirds.

Then the ship will continue on to Cabo San Lucas where the Pacific Ocean and the Sea of Cortez meet, an area of spectacular cliffs and scenic wonders.

When you go north into the Sea of Cortez after exploring Cabo San Lucas, you will come to the Gorda Banks. You will see humpback whales here. Sea lions in untold numbers will glisten on the rocks and swim near Los Islotes and later, on Isla Esperitu Santo, Audubon members will enjoy the many species of birds.

On to La Paz and while the ship spends the next week in the Sea of Cortez you will see fin whales, an occasional blue whale, and on land, the turquoise lizard. At Isla Pedro Martir you will explore the nesting areas of blue-footed boobies and brown boobies. These are rather stupid birds, but they let humans come in very close to their nests and are a photographer's delight.

As your journey ends, you will disembark in Loreto and fly home via Los Angeles. A thoroughly fascinating journey surrounded by the comforts of civilization while on board your ship!

To book see your travel agent who can book it for you at no additional cost, or —

Write or call:
>Special Expeditions, Inc.
>720 Fifth Avenue
>New York, NY 10019
>(212)765-7740

Cost: expensive
Fitness rating: moderate

BAJA EXPEDITIONS

Other companies offer tours by sea to the same area. If you have only a week's free time, for approximately half the expenditure of Sven Olof Lindblad's Special Expeditions, a company called Baja Expeditions offers adventures in which you are an active participant.

For sixteen years, Baja Expeditions has been exploring the Sea of Cortez, inspired by Steinbeck's *Log From the Sea of Cortez*. Their brochure states that they "have explored nearly every corner of Baja, by boat, kayak, skiff, muleback, on foot and on bicycle; by small planes and hot air balloons; under the sea and upon it." That sounds comprehensive.

Several of their one-week trips are centered

around whale watching during the months of the mass migration. Their ships, the *M.V. Don Jose* and *Baja Explorador*, each hold sixteen passengers and an eight- to ten-member crew. The atmosphere aboard is casual. Bath facilities are shared, which could be a disadvantage. There is a naturalist on board and a good library. The dining room features food with a Mexican touch, freshly caught fish and fruits and vegetables.

If you enjoy scuba diving, this company offers a variety of experiences in June and from July to November. In the Sea of Cortez you will see over 300 species of reef fish.

For more information, call your travel agent or —

Write or call:
> Baja Expeditions
> 2625 Garnet Ave.
> San Diego, CA 92109
> (619)581-3311

SEA ECOLOGY ADVENTURES

When I was off the coast of Baja California with a group of people about seven years ago, we traveled in a small ship that was designed primarily as a deep-sea fishing vessel. The itinerary was from San Diego and we spent several days exploring islands in the Pacific Ocean off the west side of Baja. Islas Todo Santos, Isla San Marin, Isla San Geronimo and the bigger Isla de Guadalupe were traversed and photographed.

It was a budget operation with only two bathrooms on board, and these waters were rougher than you would encounter in the Sea of Cortez. A Transderm Scop patch behind my ear changed every three days saved me and rescued a young woman who had been very seasick. These waters can be notoriously rough on the Pacific side of Baja California. Queen Elizabeth, as you may recall, was going to sail up from Cabo San Lucas in her royal yacht to meet with President Reagan, but flew instead when a storm struck. Her valiant crew brought up the ship without Her Royal Highness or Prince Philip on board.

But, despite the rough seas, this trip can also be thrilling. On San Miguel Island there are nearly 3,000 fur seals. We could clamber over fairly level ground to get in quite close to photograph the colonies. Two rolls of film later we were all saturated by the vision of so many seal pups, but their antics and noises were endearing.

Another day was spent exploring Isla (Island) Guadalupe with its huge colony of ugly elephant seals. Over 40,000 are now in this region after being almost extinct earlier in this century when only nine were believed still alive in the entire world. It is one of the great success stories in modern times regarding a once endangered species.

The males are immense, as big as trucks, and weigh between 6,000 to 8,000 pounds. Each giant male has a harem of many females, and he has to protect himself from the younger males off the coast who want to be the new king of the roost. Fights between males are noisy and frequent and their long ugly proboscises emit horrible fighting sounds. But the babies are cute and resemble little puppies with their big brown eyes.

Another thrill along these waters is the frequent sightings of whales on their migration, and we saw dozens of them. At night the dolphins appeared phosphorescent and were intriguing to watch as they cavorted just off the bow of our ship.

If I had had more funds and more time, this same company would have taken us to Magdalena Bay where we could have visited the breeding area of the California gray whale.

If you have good sea legs and enjoy sailing on the open sea, this company can provide a great learning experience. We were fortunate to have a brilliant marine biologist on board whose field of expertise was the Cetaceans (whales) and a young botanist working on his Ph.D. in San Diego.

Write or call:
    H and M Landings
    2803 Emerson Street
    San Diego, CA 92106
    (619) 222-1144
Cost: moderate
Fitness rating: strenuous
Wheelchair access: no

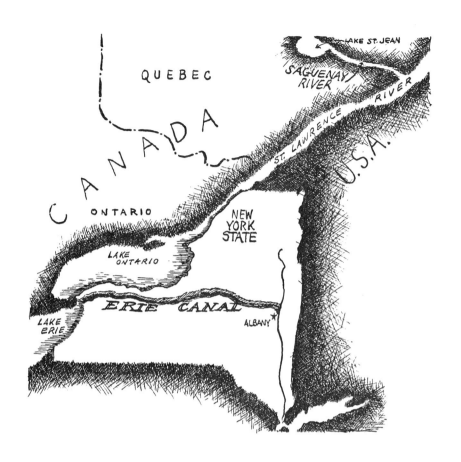

FROM THE ERIE CANAL TO SAGUENAY

Jim and June Duncan recently returned from a cruise on board the *New Shoreham ll.* Navigating the Erie Canal aboard American Canadian Caribbean Line's *New Shoreham ll* turned out to be a very different experience from the famous folk song every American child used to sing. They went further than the fifteen miles covered by that old mule named Sal, but at one point it was like the refrain, "Low bridge, everybody down, low bridge, for we're going through a town."

American Canadian Caribbean Line has the only passenger ships that can navigate the Erie Canal because of the canal's low bridges. Jim and June watched in amazement as the pilot house on their ship was lowered down one entire deck in height so that the ship could inch its way under those low bridges! A crew waited on shore to help with this complicated process.

The Duncans are a young retired couple in their 60s who enjoy boating and Shakespeare. Perhaps because they own their own boat, which they take out many weekends into San Francisco Bay, they did not want the glitzy cruise experience which requires the man to dress formally for dinner. They enjoyed the informal atmosphere on this ship which holds only 80 passengers, and they liked the one serving, open seating policy. This allowed them to mingle with other guests at all of the meals and become acquainted with many interesting people. If you've ever suffered through an entire week of cruising assigned to a table where you have been saddled with a loud boor and are not permitted to change your dining companions, you will see this flexibility as a great advantage.

As the ship journeyed through locks, the crew had to climb up a narrow little ladder set in the walls of the locks which appeared to be 40 feet in height.

The crew then helped the ship avoid hitting the walls as it went through the locks, as the water rises rapidly, causing turbulence. (In the reverse direction, the water lowers, of course!)

From the West Coast, passengers fly into Providence, Rhode Island, and stay overnight, for an added expense, at the comfortable Marriott Hotel. The travelers are then picked up at the hotel the next morning at 8 A.M. for the beginning of their adventure.

ACCL has two sister ships, the *New Shoreham II* and the *Caribbean Prince*, which follow back-to-back itineraries on this routing between the Erie Canal and the Saguenay River in Canada from early June until the middle of September.

From Warren, Rhode Island the cruise ship sailed through Narragansett Bay and along the shores of New England as it neared New York. Reaching Long Island Sound, passengers arrived in the New York harbor at daybreak. As the ship cruised up Hudson Bay it passed many famous mansions and West Point, eventually coming to the Erie Canal. From here they traveled through a series of locks until the ship reached Lake Ontario and the area of Thousand Islands.

In this area they took a smaller day cruise for awhile on a smaller ship. Many homes are located on these islands, which are sometimes so small that there is just one home on the entire island. Some of these island homes looked very idyllic with tall pines and shubbery protecting the owner's privacy. Others had foot bridges or car bridges leading to other islands. One such bridge was built by the original owner, and halfway across he marked the division between America and Canada. He used to joke and say if he and his wife ever had an argument he could just leave the country!

As they cruised the St. Lawrence Seaway, they spent two nights in Montreal and two nights in Quebec, long enough to explore these two cities which have French as their first language. In Quebec, they saw stately buildings with the old copper roofs that turned into a burnished turquoise color as the buildings aged.

The final destination on this voyage was the Saguenay River, a fiord which is in an area of great rugged beauty. This river is where the Beluga whale breeds. Appropriately the passengers disembarked for one last time on the shore of the Bay of Eternity. After exploring these distant shores, the passengers returned to their ship which transported them back to Montreal.

A bus with air conditioning took the passengers then by land back to Warren, Rhode Island, where they caught their flights back to their home states.

The Duncans thoroughly enjoyed their cruise and would like to travel again on the same cruiseline.

This cruise company offers some other exciting itineraries. There are four fall foliage cruise tours through late September and all of October. Then a repositioning cruise to Florida follows. During the winter there are voyages around the Florida Everglades, from Belize to Rio Dulce for sun worshippers and snorkelers, as a way to escape from the cold up north for those aboard the *Caribbean Prince,* while those passengers on the *New Shoreham II* enjoy cruising around the Virgin Islands. Book with your travel agent, or —

Write or call:
American Canadian Caribbean Line, Inc.
P.O. Box 36
Warren, R.I. 02885
(401)247-0955
Cost: varies according to type of cabin or stateroom desired, but begins in the range of inexpensive
Fitness rating: easy
Wheelchair access: inquire directly

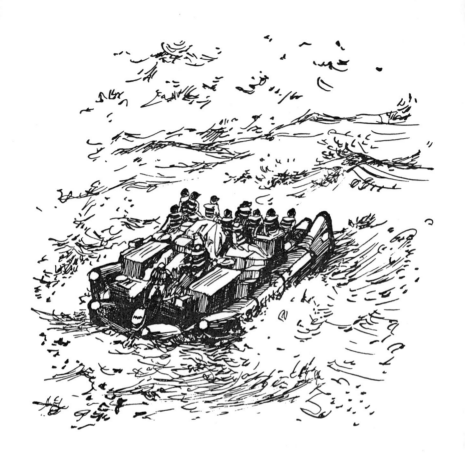

RIVER RAFTING

WESTERN RIVER EXPEDITIONS

Have you ever been served flaming baked Alaska by a bronzed young man clad only in a tee shirt with a tuxedo motif on it and a pair of black shorts? That is your treat on the last evening of your rafting adventure with Western River Expeditions. (The baked Alaska, not the unobtainable bronzed young man.)

My friends and clients, Ray Fontaine and Karen Wilson-Fontaine, were struck by the incongruity of gourmet meals served with a flair after an action-packed day of rafting on the Grand Canyon's Colorado River. You may have the impression of "roughing it" during the day when you are sprayed with water or are gazing up at the awesome beauty of the Grand Canyon, but you do not have to cook your own flapjacks over a campfire, nor do you have to gather twigs for that fire.

Buffet breakfasts are followed by smorgasbord lunches where you create your own "Dagwood" sandwich from a tempting array of selections. Each night has barbecued or Dutch-oven prepared main dishes, salads, rolls and desserts.

Food is not the lure on these excursions, however. The joy of a vacation spent in the area of one of America's most scenic wonders is the reason for the journey. You will see the Grand Canyon from a perspective that few others have. The grandeur is magnificent and as you gaze upwards 1,000 feet at the various hues and colors of the towering gorge above you, awestruck by its beauty, its immensity will overwhelm you.

The six-day rafting adventure on the Colorado River is filled with experiences very different from what the city dweller encounters at home. The thrills and excitement engendered on such a trip drive away all of your usual worries. Here, the danger comes not from a driver behind the wheel on a crowded modern freeway, but from the whitewater rapids, from nature itself, and your first lesson after clambering onto the raft is how to hold the ropes safely.

Riding over the Lava Falls Rapids, the most dangerous set of rapids on the Colorado River, is not for the faint-hearted. But if you have been a thrill-seeker all of your life and still enjoy roller coaster rides, this would be exhilarting for you. All you have to do physically is to hold on tight to the ropes in front and in back of you, close your eyes, and pray. Let the young and experienced guide do the rest.

You will have five days of running smaller rapids, of mastering safety instructions, of enjoying daily thrills, before you reach the Lava Falls. There have been high jinks as well. On the Fontaine's trip, a single raft managed to get a half hour ahead of the others, and suddenly, going under a nature bridge, their "friends" doused their raft with buckets of water from above. Since they were already drenched from running the rapids, a little more water only called for another prank in return.

Discover the beauty of the Grand Canyon from the river with the rafts from Western River Expeditions. The rafts are unsinkable and are considered to be the safest crafts on the river. When you see this raft springing over a rapid, it resembles an undulating caterpillar or an inchworm from a distance, because it bends as it goes over the rapids.

Six different climatic zones are traversed in the 188-mile journey and you see many wildflowers. There are always some flowers blooming throughout the year because of these dramatic changes in the climate.

One sleeps in sleeping bags and gazes upwards at the magnificent cliffs. The cliffs can resemble well-known areas of the world. One such formation is called the "Bridge of Sighs," after the structure of that name in Venice.

As you journey on the raft, you are following the path Major Powell explored over a hundred years ago in 1869. The Colorado River emerges from Lake Powell and is usually a beautiful green color. As in Bandelier National Park, there are many deserted cliff dwellings where native Indians lived centuries ago. During the six days spent here, some of these ancient homes will be explored by the group.

While you slumber in your sleeping bags, in tents if you wish, at dawn your breakfast is being prepared. It is not quite breakfast in bed, but the rich aromas of bacon frying, coffee brewing, and the sound of flapjacks being flipped, will bring you out of your warm nest.

Even the gentle moments on this trip call for caution, however. It looks idyllic to shower under a waterfall, yet Deer Creek Falls is so deep and rapid that people stand only in its mist to cool off on a hot day. To stand directly beneath it would be painful because of the force of the water falling from such a height.

Havasu Creek is a blue green, warm 70 degrees, and usually at least four hours are spent relaxing here in the many pools.

At the end of the trip everyone felt it had been a very exciting and invigorating journey. "A good cure for urban depression," said one young woman. People came from all over the world to experience the Grand Canyon in this exciting adventure and they formed bonds of friendship, going away with unforgettable memories.

The Fontaines love river rafting, and Karen stated that there is something so exhilarating, so primeval about this particular trip that she would be happy to return to this area for the same adventure each year. One of the people on their raft was over 65, and that participant took a more active role in the explorations than many of the younger ones.

To book this trip, see your travel agent or —

Write or call:

    Western River Expeditions
    7258 Racquet Club Drive
    Salt Lake City, UT 84121
    (801) 942-6669

Cost: expensive
Fitness rating: moderate

A Note of Caution

In their brochure, Western River Expeditions states, "We feel that your Western River expedition is safer than a week's vacation in your car . . . however, you should recognize that there is an element of risk in any adventure, sport or activity associated with the outdoors."

The brochure recommends that the participant take out additional medical insurance to cover himself during that adventure. Trip insurance is often also advisable. I personally have known three people who have incurred injuries while rafting (in every case, their feet were braced under straps in the raft). Therefore, it is best to enter into these adventures with your eyes wide open. I would strongly suggest that you find out about the safety record of a company before booking an adventure.

Western River Expeditions does exercise caution. If Lava Falls Rapids, the one that gives the rafting participants the greatest thrills, is too turbulent because of uncertain weather conditions, the young experienced guides will alter the itinerary. You may find yourself walking around these rapids or on an alternate route.

With this same company, if you have never experienced white water rafting before, you might want to sign up for a tamer version. The four-day rafting trip begins below the mighty Lava Falls and is preceded by a day spent on a ranch. An old-fashioned western day of horseback riding and watching real cowboys is followed by three days of rafting in gentler water. Although there are rapids on this trip, they are do not appear so spectacular or dangerous. This looks like a good trip for the older adult who wants to enjoy the beauty of this scenic wonderland in complete safety.

RAFTING DOWN THE MENDENHALL RIVER

I have thoroughly enjoyed rafting on the Mendenhall River out of Juneau, Alaska. We were first driven out to view the mighty Mendenhall Glacier, one of the world's most photographed wonders. Areas of brilliant blue were evidence of recent calving which occurs when huge chunks of ice break off. Boulders of newly freed glacial ice were tumbling about in the river.

We were given big yellow raincoats and tall rubber boots before we climbed into the rafts. Each raft held eight to ten people. Our experienced boatman gave us a natural history lesson as we floated along past forests, rustic cabins, and mountain peaks. We could see fish in the clear glacial water. Three moose sauntered out of the forest and swam in front of us. Eagles flow overhead.

At times our raft would pick up momentum as we glided over gentle rapids. Our hair was soaked and we laughed with glee, uncaring about our appearance, enjoying the sensation.

All too soon, we scrambled ashore and tasted a wild alcoholic blend called "Mendenhall Madness," made cold with the blue ice form the glacier. Smoked salmon, squaw bread and reindeer sausage were served. Apple cider cheered those who were thirsty, but did not wish to imbibe. It was a morning of adventure none of us would ever forget. If you visit Juneau, try this Mendenhall Glacier Float trip.

It will appeal to all of your senses!
Book while in Juneau, or —

Write or call:
Alaska Travel Adventures
9085-TA Glacier Highway, Suite 204
Juneau, AK 99801
(907) 789-0052

Cost: inexpensive
Fitness rating: easy

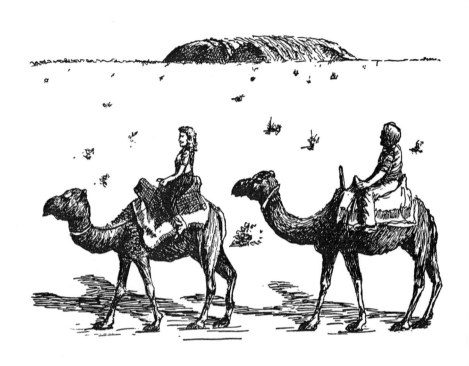

CAMELS, CROCODILES AND FAIRY PENGUINS

If you would like to ride a camel or come close to a crocodile in Crocodile Dundee's land "down under," then Brendan Tours offers an exciting tour for those of you who wish to see many of the wild things in their natural setting.

The group flies into Melbourne, Australia, relaxes that first day, and then you begin to explore this city which is very European in flavor. Visit Captain Cook's Cottage in the Fitzroy Gardens, a historic mansion, and the Botanical Gardens, where one can feed the swans and see some rare plants indigenous to Australia.

What I most remember about Melbourne is the city's unique way of nabbing motorists who are speeding or who run a red light. A camera is located at the intersections and if someone zooms through a red light, a photograph is sent out to the person along with a polite letter and a fine. Caught red-handed!

Australia's justice system is more like the British and at certain times of day it is entertaining to see men leap out of their cars, grab their briefcases, and hustle off to court carrying their black robes, white wigs slightly askew on their heads.

FAIRY PENGUINS, ALICE SPRINGS AND AYRES ROCK

From Melbourne do take the optional drive out to see the fairy penguins waddle in by the thousands at twilight. Dress warmly, for this mass exodus takes place on a rugged, windy area of the sea coast. The penguins are tiny as they emerge from the sea and scurry along, ignoring the humans lined up to see them. The penguins glisten in the moonlight and come in very close to the viewers. Flash on your camera is strictly prohibited. No one should startle these little fellows.

Flying out the next day, this particular tour takes

the travelers to Alice Springs. You will visit the Outback, see the historic Telegraph Station and visit the Royal Flying Doctor Service. That evening's dinner will be a barbecue served in the bush. As you munch on damper bread, drink billy tea, and enjoy a good beef dinner, you will hear tales about the Aborigines. Your hotel is not a bed roll on the ground, however, but a first class Sheraton.

By bus the group drives on and is taken to Virginia Camel Farm. Here you can ride on the camels and be photographed while you are enjoying this camel ride in the famous Australian Outback. The evening finds you photographing the world famous Ayers Rock, the largest monolith in the world — two miles long and 1099 feet high. Because it is sacred to the aboriginal tribes, visitors don't stay right here in Uluru Park, but some twelve miles away.

The next morning you will explore Ayers Rock in more depth, learning more about the aboriginal culture, and you will visit some of the caves near the base of the rock.

A flight on to Darwin lands the travelers in Kakadu National Park. Cruise on a boat and see the crocodiles and unique bird life in this region.

The next day will be one in which travelers can examine aboriginal drawings on rocks and visit archaelogical sites. Then a day is spent exploring Darwin and everyone flies on that evening to Cairns.

A day is spent on Green Island (see page 130), enjoying the Great Barrier Reef and the Underwater Observatory.

On the tenth day the group flies to Sydney, a modern and vibrant city. The bus takes the group across a bridge and to Ku-ring-gai Chase National Park to view kangaroos which you can pet and feed. A Captain Cook cruise follows, with lunch on board. The rest of the day is free. A suggestion is to see an opera that evening at the Sydney Opera House, but this must be booked when you are first arranging the tour back in the states. It is very difficult to procure opera tickets after you arrive in Sydney.

If you are a single person, tell your travel agent you wish to share. If Brendan can match you up with another single traveler, the single surcharge will be returned to you. To book this twelve-day tour, call your travel agent, or —

Write or call:
  Brendan Tours
  15137 Califa Street
  Van Nuys, CA 91411
  Fax: (818) 902-9876
Cost: expensive
Fitness rating: moderate
Wheelchair access: not on this tour, but Brendan has other tours of Australia and New Zealand which might be suitable. It requests that handicapped people inform their travel agent and then that they travel with someone who can help and who will be responsible for the traveler in the wheelchair.

TAKE A CAMEL TO LUNCH

Frontier Tours offers packages which feature excursions to visit the Frontier Camel Farm, out of Alice Springs, some 280 miles away from Ayers Rock. You can take a camel on an hour's riding adventure along the sandy area of Todd River after breakfast at the camel farm or before lunch and dinner, which are served at Chateau Hornsby Winery. Breakfast is the most reasonably priced of the three choices. The cost once you are in the region is reasonable; the trick is to get there — an expensive flight into Alice Springs is needed first.

Or would you rather "Spend a Night with a Camel?" This is a new offering in 1991 by Adventure Center. In this adventure, participants are driven 90 miles from Alice Springs. After arriving in Western MacDonnell Ranges, they'll enjoy a barbecue in the bush and become acquainted with one another.

Then they'll mount their camels, ride all afternoon and camp out for the night, enjoying the stars in the Southern Hemisphere.

On the second day, the adventurers will ride on, following trails along the Finke River to Glen Helen Lodge. Here they will spend the night in solid comfort and enjoy dinner at Cloudy's Restaurant. Famous in this region for its good food, residents of Alice Springs have been known to drive the 80 miles to enjoy dinner out here. On the third day after breakfast, the group will return to Alice Springs.

Book with a travel agent, or —

Write or call:
> Adventure Center
> 1311 63rd Street #200
> Emeryville, CA 94608
> (800) 228-8747 in California
> (800) 227-8747 outside California

Cost: inexpensive

Fitness rating: strenuous for someone like myself who aches after getting off of a horse!

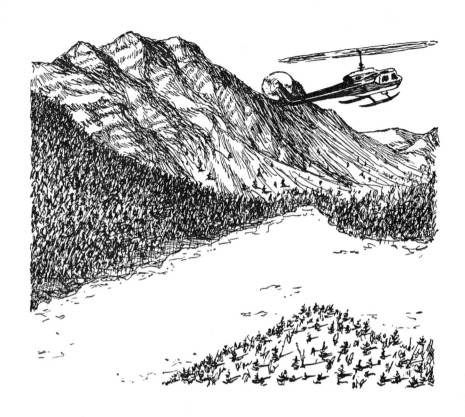

HELI-EXPLORING IN THE CARIBOOS OR BUGABOOS

Heli-hiking has been honed to perfection with Tauck Tours. It can be the basis for a summer vacation in the Canadian Rockies that you'll never forget.

Tauck Tours is noted in the travel industry for providing first class quality tours for the United States and Canada. It is a company which puts quality and service ahead of mass marketing. Intentionally it keeps its groups down to 35 to 44 with the same tour guide with the group at all times. If you've ever been on one of those inexpensive bus tours in Europe where 59 people are crammed into one bus, you'll appreciate the difference a smaller group can make.

Heli-exploring or heli-hiking is an exciting way to explore inaccessible areas where there are no roads. Now you no longer have to park your car at a vista point and stare up at these magnificent Canadian Rockies. Now you can fly in a helicopter to near the top of those peaks and explore a region with fields of alpine wild flowers, see pristine lakes and take prize-winning photographs. After you have explored one area for an hour or so, the helicopter returns and takes its ten passengers on to another unexplored wilderness area. This is where you may enjoy a picnic by a quiet mountain stream before continuing to explore at your own pace.

My friend and pupil, Margaret Kinnicutt, excited my imagination with her descriptions of this tour. When she was in her early 70s, she traveled with Tauck to this region. She had worried that she might not be able to climb up into the helicopter, but it proved to be easy. Sixty percent of those going on these tours are over 50, and the most recent brochure states, "With heli-exploring, age is no barrier. In the past ten years, we have catered to persons from 8 to 85."

The groups are organized by individuals' descriptions of their physical capabilities. If older people wish to merely stroll along level areas without any rugged climbing, that is where the helicopter transports them. If the younger or more physically active, which could be of any age, want a climbing challenge, the helicopter takes them nearer to that goal. The choice is up to the participant.

Here is a description of one of Tauck's nine-day, eight-night tours. After you arrive in Calgary, the tour is all inclusive. Breakfast and dinner are included daily. If, however, you fly in from the West Coast, you might have to overnight at the Westin Hotel at an additional expense because the tour departs in the early afternoon of the first day of the tour. From Calgary you travel to Banff Springs Hotel, that enormous hotel which boasts of championship golf courses, but which is better known for the spectacular natural beauty of the surrounding countryside. The next morning you will enjoy a rafting adventure on the Bow River.

On the third day the group heads for Lake Louise, passing gorges formed by glaciers and snow-covered mountain peaks, and then visits Kicking Horse Pass and later the Continental Divide. The Chateau Lake Louise, which resembles a tall castle, is your hotel that night. Every room Tauck has reserved has a glorious view of Lake Louise.

Then on to the Banff-Jasper Highway the next morning, which has waterfalls and lakes along this road located in the Canadian National Parks. If you're lucky, you'll see deer, brown bears, big horned sheep and moose. That night and the next will be spent at Jasper Park Lodge, set near another beautiful lake. Here again, golfers may want to play nine or eighteen holes on the free day that follows your arrival. Horseback riding is offered along trails, hiking or swimming is available.

Then the real adventure begins. On the sixth day you pack only a few overnight items in the small bag Tauck provides, leaving most of your belongings behind in your suitcases which will be stored at Jasper Park Lodge.

You now drive to the helicopter area where, in groups of eight to ten, you will be flown up high into the Cariboo Mountains and taken to the Cariboo Lodge which will be your home for the next two nights. After everyone has assembled here and the first arrivals have explored the area, the helicopter may be free to give everyone at least one more heli-exploring adventure that day — a mountain valley meadow strewn with colorful wild flowers — before you feel hunger pangs for dinner at the lodge.

The entire next day is spent heli-hiking or heli-exploring. So much to be explored and enjoyed! You will be one of the rare few in the world to visit these remote alpine meadows. Wild flowers that bloom in April and May in California are blooming up here in this brief summertime of long days and shortened nights. Indian paintbrush, bluebells, fields of lupin, waterfalls and views of breathtaking splendor are yours to enjoy.

Then it's the anticlimatic last day spent bringing you back to civilization, to Edmonton and one last hotel before departing for home, armed with memories and with new and lasting friendships.

As long as you can climb up two 20-inch steps into the helicopter and can withstand the altitude of 10,000 feet, this trip could bring you great joy and the satisfaction of feeling you have conquered new vistas.

To book, see your travel agent to arrange the lowest possible air fare. Tauck prefers working with agents and its brochure only states its address:

Write:
      Tauck Tours, Inc.
      P.O. Box 5027
      Westport, Ct 06881

Cost: expensive

Fitness rating: moderate to strenuous. The pace is up to you.

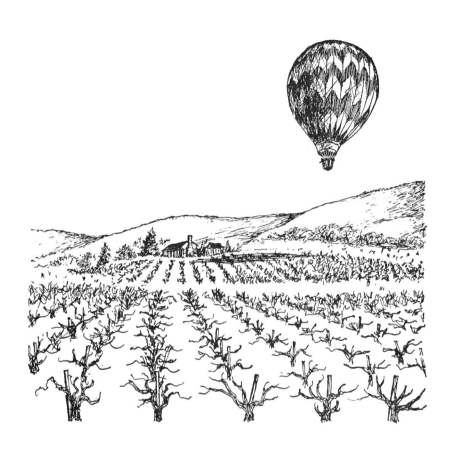

BALLOONING IN CALIFORNIA

You don't have to travel halfway around the world to enjoy an unusual adventure. It is not necessary to travel far to enjoy a weekend or a day that is extraordinary. Every state offers exciting activities which may not be found elsewhere.

Since I reside in California, I'll tell you about two ballooning adventures which are offered in our state. I know that I have not mentioned ballooning over the wine country in Australia, which is a beautiful and exciting adventure, but ballooning is also offered in our own wine growing regions of California, and it may be possible close to you.

BALLOONING IN THE
NAPA VALLEY WINE COUNTRY

Many of my friends and pupils have gone hot air ballooning over the vineyards of the Napa Valley. Some have had to make repeated attempts and spent several enjoyable weekends in that region waiting for the weather to be ideal for the adventure. No expert balloonist will take a group up if there are high winds or rain.

One of my pupils, Beth Brewster, wrote of her balloon ride in the Napa Valley for her 65th birthday:

"Talk about a day to remember! We sailed around above the lava cliffs and green vineyards of that beautiful spot, with sixteen other brilliant balloons. All the passengers waved every time we got close enough, and it seemed that our dream world was full of happy people. I didn't care if we never came down!

"The weather was exactly right, and the winds heard my prayer for a long ride. The contracted hour passed in a flash, of course; but then every time we passed over the landing field, the wind changed direction, and we'd have to circle out and around, and try again. It took a couple of hours before we swung low enough for the ground crew to catch us and bring us to earth. After that, the champagne breakfast was anti-climatic.

"I plan to do it again when I'm 75."

An adventurous spirit!

Write or call:
> Napa Valley Balloons, Inc.
> P.O. Box 2860
> Yountville, CA 94599
> (800) 253-2224

Cost: moderate

Fitness rating: easy, but you must stand for an hour or two, holding onto the basket

PROFESSOR MULDOON
AND HIS HOT AIR BALLOON

For years my own mother had said, "I've ridden on a camel, on a mule in Greece, on a horse in Pennsylvania as I was growing up, but I've never been up in a balloon. How I would love to do that."

So, on her birthday when she was in her early 80s, I took her before dawn one morning to rendezvous with Professor Muldoon and his hot air balloon at the Livermore airport.

In early September, it was still dark when we first assembled along with another friend of ours who had just turned 80. Three others soon joined us. They were all anticipating ballooning over the vineyards that surround Livermore. Both Wente Brothers and Concannon Wineries are located in this valley, as well as several smaller ones.

Unfortunately, it was too windy here and we drove

inland to Tracy, a 20-minute drive over the Altamont Pass, past thousands of modern wind mills churning busily in the early morning wind, creating electric energy power, enough for many homes and businesses.

At last we came to the tiny airstrip outside of Tracy and the balloon was inflated — a big brilliant sphere of reds, pinks, greens, and blues in undulating patterns — a magic sphere which was soon to be like a magic carpet bearing Mother and others up into the clouds.

There were openings in the large basket big enough for toe holds, and everyone clambered in. Down on the ground, I was with the landlubbers in the truck that chased after the balloon.

It grew tinier and tinier as it rose, and for a time it was difficult to see at all, but as it floated towards earth an hour later, a dog on the ranch where Professor Muldoon has landing privileges, came rushing out and barked at the strange object as it came down, swaying gently and making whooshing noises. Everyone aboard was grinning widely and champagne spilled enthusiastically into everyone's glass as a special pronouncement was made, congratulating everyone.

The hills and farmlands below the passengers had been like a kaleidoscope of changing patterns. The streams had appeared like tiny silver ribbons in the early morning sunlight.

It was truly a morning to remember. Professor

Muldóon is a charming theatrical type of character with an impressive safety record. He enhances the journey and makes it fun for everyone.

It would have been a beautiful trip over the vineyards of the Livermore Valley where so many prize-winning white wines are created, but flexibility helped in the spirit of adventure. By substituting another farming area, they passed over hundreds of Holstein dairy cattle, over fields of ripening corn, acres of melons, and miles of cultivated fruit trees. In the spring, that might even be the more beautiful journey when those thousands of trees are blossoming.

Flexibilty is the key to success in many an adventure — flexibility and an open mind.

Write or call:
   Professor Muldoon's Hot Air Balloon
   P.O. Box 667
   Pleasanton, Ca. 94566
   (800)822-3333
Cost: moderate
Fitness rating: easy

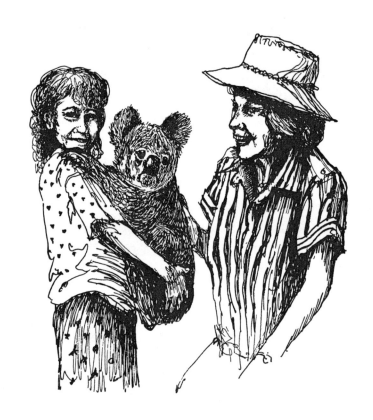

ADVENTURES WITH YOUR GRANDCHILDREN

It is a joy to share your pleasures with others whom you love, and you might want to take your grandchildren along with you on one of your adventures as you explore the world. I have escorted groups of all ages, and the intergenerations are delightful. You might want to spoil one at a time when he or she has reached a milestone in life, such as a graduation from high school, or you might want two or three to accompany you. Then you might wish to have the three generations along! On a cruise ship recently a couple were celebrating their golden wedding anniversary. Their entire family came. It was a week-long party for about 23 family members.

We can not all be so generous, but holidays shared are a good time to really become better acquainted with one's family and with one's grandchildren.

SUGGESTIONS FOR VACATION ADVENTURES

After the children have demonstrated good swimming skills they would enjoy river rafting if they are at least seven or eight years old, at the safe levels of 1 or 11. You do not wish to place them in danger. Check the safety record of the company.

The family can rent an entire houseboat here in the United States, such as is found on California's Lake Shasta or the Sacramento River delta. There is something for everyone on these boats. If you enjoy sunbathing, swimming, diving, fishing or exploring, or have a yen to be a navigator, now is your chance.

Barging in France is fun when the family rents a small "bare bones" barge. Some hold just six to eight passengers and you can prepare your own meals on board or dine out in the villages along the canals, and just prepare light breakfasts and lunches on board.

Rent a houseboat in England. Float on the Norfolk Broads for a week past picturesque towns far from the major highways. You'll have a chance to explore villages and mingle with other English-speaking families in a way you could not on a regular tour.

Photo safaris to almost anywhere are delightful. Treat your grandchild to an inexpensive camera and train him to see selectively.

A tour to your country of origin or to the country of your family's heritage would be very meaningful, particularly if you still have relatives living in that country. One pupil of mine made at least eight trips to Wales, the land of his parents. He discovered first and second cousins still living and plunged into genealogy. His entire family was drawn into this enthusiastic search.

A visit to any ancient walled city in Europe is fascinating for your grandchildren. Children of all ages love to clamber over the older portions of the walls and explore the ramparts. Our family of three generations explored two cities together. Carcassonne, in the south of France, has never been conquered. Its historic walls are over 600 years old. We also immensely enjoyed Rothenburg in Germany. This is the city where Danny Kaye made the film classic about Hans Christian Anderson. (It was not filmed in Denmark.) We walked all around the city, peering down on its ancient buildings from the vantage point of the ramparts which encircled it. Castles in every country of Europe are often open to the public, and fascinate children of all ages.

Within major European cities you can arrange part

of each day for an activity which has wide appeal for children. My husband and I alternated between visits to art galleries and museums, which fascinated my mother and us, but then we included a treat for the youngsters.

The Zoo

Zoos abroad are often better than in this country unless you compare them to San Diego's. Often in Europe the animals do not seem to be behind bars, but are in clever enclosures or behind moats that minimize that caged effect.

Natural History Museums

This is a good choice for rainy days. In Europe, the exhibits are labeled in several languages, including English. When my husband attended a conference, I took the children to these museums.

Science Museums

A tour of a museum which inspires future scientists and engineers such as our Smithsonian Air and Space Museum in Washington, D.C. or Das Deutsches Museum in Munich, Germany is always a fascinating pastime.

Toy Museums

Many major cities, such as London, have one.

The Great Outdoors

Another treat would be to share your love of the out-of-doors with your grandchild. Share a visit to our national parks. Audubon members often take their children or grandchildren along on their day excursions. It is great exercise for everyone, and their eyes may spot that rare bird before you do. Give them the gift of your respect for our wildlife and for our wilderness areas.

In Hawaii recently, we saw all of the generations enjoying themselves. Perhaps the entire family had a vacation rental of a condo together. We saw parents and grandparents helping their children and grandchildren to snorkel and to feed the fish frozen green peas. It was heartwarming to see. It is one way for everyone to enjoy themselves, particularly if the generations are scattered all over America. To assemble once a year and vacation together is a joyful event.

You will be building memories for your grandchildren, memories that they will never forget and that you will always cherish.

For arrangements for the vacations abroad, see your favorite travel agent, who can arrange for any type of trip you might wish to share with your grandchild.

GRANDTRAVEL

This new company carefully arranges very expensive tours for grandparents and their grandchildren. It will cooperate with your travel agent and concoct a worry-free vacation for you. Although it is available for children of any age, its brochure states that children between the ages of 7 and 14 seem to take the keenest pleasure in the activities offered. You are provided with an escort at all times, and certain activities are planned just for the grandparents and certain others just for the children, so that the needs of all ages are met. Send for their tempting catalog of adventures in and outside North America.

Write or call:

Grandtravel
6900 Wisconsin Ave.
Suite 706
Chevy Chase, MD 20815
(301) 986-0890

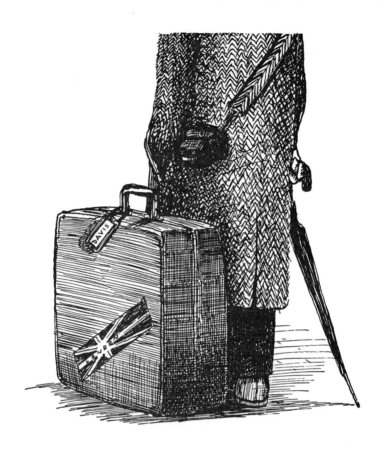

TRAVELING SINGLE

If you are newly single, or have always been, and feel uncomfortable about traveling alone, many people in the travel industry can offer you an enjoyable, safe, and economical traveling experience.

Traveling as a single can be expensive. Many cruise lines charge a person who wishes to book a single cabin 160% of the cost per person for a double occupany. For more expensive cabins, the charge is often 200%. Instead of paying $7,000 for a twelve-day cruise and enjoying a cabin with a friend or spouse, you might have to pay $14,000 as a single!

There are exceptions to these kinds of penalties. At least one cruise line, Royal Cruise Line, which thoroughly pampers its guests, will arrange a cabin-mate for you according to your age group, smoking or nonsmoking preference and sex. In the twelve lower categories, you may request a share through your travel agent, and if one is not found for you, you will not have to pay any additional fee. A very generous arrangement.

Traveling alone can be very costly for you on a land tour, also. A single supplement charge for you to have a room to yourself on a European tour can range from $350 to over $1000.

However, there are certain tour operators who realize the hardship this places on those who travel alone, and these companies arrange roommates for you, according to your approximate age, your sex, and whether you are a smoker or a nonsmoker.

For my own tours or for the college I am always happy to arrange roommates for my participants and often have a party prior to our departure to introduce everyone.

TRAFALGAR

One tour company which reaches out to the single traveler is Trafalgar, which offers a roommate matching service. Its brochure states, "If you are traveling alone and don't mind sharing, Trafalgar will arrange for you to share a twin room with someone of the same sex. If we don't find a partner for you, you still don't have to pay the single supplement. Tell this to your travel agent when you book." One drawback to a Trafalgar tour is that during high season on their European tours you may find yourself in a big bus which seats 59 people.

BRENDAN TOURS

As mentioned elsewhere, if you wish to travel to New Zealand, Brendan Tours offers to match you up with a rommmate on fully escorted tours. You need to pay the single supplement prior to departure, but Brenden makes every effort to secure a roommate for you. If you are compatible, and stay as roommates throughout the tour, you are refunded the extra money you sent as a single.

SINGLEWORLD

At least two other companies cater to singles. Singleworld is now in its 34th year. It offers tours and cruises. There are "under 35" age group trips and those planned for "all ages." Singleworld states that it is not a lonely hearts club, and for a non-refundable fee of $25 per person per year, one is sent a newsletter four times a year telling the members of new destinations and new tours. All of these tours can be booked with your favorite travel agent. The least expensive costs for their cruises are for quads — a cabin which holds four people. The organization also arranges double occupancy if you wish. For further information —

Write:

> Gramercy's Singleworld
> 401 Theodore Fremd Avenue
> Rye, NY 10580

CLASSIC SINGLES NETWORK

For elegant travel as a single, Olson Travel, Cartan and Conner Tours offer "Classic Singles Network." These tours are operated in Europe, England and Ireland, Egypt, the Orient, America, Canada and Hawaii. They encourage you to fill out an application which you may produre from your travel agent which shows your interests and general age group. If you request a share, and they are unable to secure a roommate for you on your first choice of a tour, they will suggest another tour where there is a share available. If you do not wish this change, then you pay the single supplement.

These are first class tours and often the groups are limited to 27 or 28 participants, thus assuring you of more personalized service and a smaller bus, a big plus in European travel where the most historic areas have narrow streets better suited to a horse and carriage than to anything larger.

For more information, see your travel agent or —

Write:

> First Family of Travel
> Classic Singles Network
> P.O. Box 92734
> Los Angeles, CA 90009

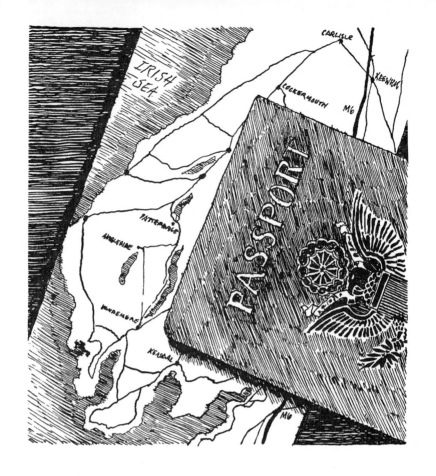

HELPFUL HINTS

Use a Travel Agent

Herb Caen, the famous *San Francisco Chronicle* columnist, wrote about one of his own trips from London: "This trip must have been planned by a maniac and it was. Caenfucius say: Man who acts as own travel agent has fool for client. . . if I'd been in charge of D-Day planning, the U.S. First, Third, and 29th Divisions would have landed on Omaha Beach in Nebraska."

A good travel agent can actually save you a great deal of money and it costs no more to book a tour with a travel agent than with a tour company. The travel agent can point out the differences to you in the various tours to the destination you wish to visit. One tour to Tahiti, for example, might look like it is considerably less in cost than another. When you examine it closely, the bargain tour might delete the costs of inter-island flights and all meals. Meals on your own in Tahiti are very costly, and you would probably end up spending more eventually on the "bargain" tour than for the slightly higher, all-inclusive tour.

A travel agent earns his or her commission from the supplier, from the tour company or from the airlines without any increase in cost to you, the consumer.

The agent can also coordinate all of your flights to your destination and can compare the prices of all ten carriers flying there. If you call one airline, you will get only that airline's price and a series of rules. In this era of deregulation, on November 23, 1990 there were 159 different fares between San Francisco and Los Angeles alone, 79 between Oakland and Los Angeles, and 87 between San Jose and Los Angeles! Not only is that ridiculous, but only a computerized travel agency can sort through these and find you the lowest fares.

Bucket Shops

Beware of "bucket shops" which advertise very low fares. Often the owner of such a shop is operating with only a phone number and a post office box. He may have no legitimate address and will not be bonded.

Travel agents now work with consolidators if you want the very lowest fare between two set international destinations such as New York and London, for example. However, if you miss your flight for any reason whatsoever, you may lose all of your money. It will be a nonrefundable, nonchangeable fare. Such fares lack the flexibility you may need to join a tour on the right date. You may have to accept a date for any day within a week's period to get that inexpensive ticket.

Many consolidators buy up blocks of tickets in the last month for certain flights — tickets that the airline has not been able to sell. Therefore most consolidators can not confirm flights until you are within a month of departing. Then that tour you wanted to take may be all booked up.

Bucket shops are even worse. It used to be illegal to sell tickets as they do when the industry was regulated and the public had more protection. Bucket shops have been known to abscond with your funds and not forward the money to pay for your airline flight or your hotel. Sometimes tickets are issued which other airlines will not honor.

You arrive at the airport in Amsterdam, for example. Your plane is one from the Middle East, but it is overbooked and you are not allowed to board. To fly back to the West Coast you have to pay over $1,000 one way for your ticket because no other carrier will recognize the validity of the ticket you have.

Travel Scams

Beware of travel scams which keep cropping up in new forms with new disguises. Do not give out your credit card number over the phone when you receive an out-of-state solicitation for a deal which sounds too good to be true. It probably is.

Beware of telemarketing travel scams. Congress is trying to pass legislation to protect the consumer. People lose thousands of dollars by not going through a reputable firm. One man paid $2,000 to a travel promoter. He checked later with the hotel and the airlines, and found he had never been booked. The tour office was dark. There was no answer when he tried to call. The promoter at the bucket shop had fled with his money and will victimize others in another part of the country until he is apprehended.

Reliable bonded agencies have to protect your money and place it in an escrow account.

Here is one example of a travel scam, described by Barbara Kaufman, columnist for the *Valley Times*.

"The free-ticket scam. You receive one free airline ticket if you purchase a second airline ticket; however, you have to buy a 'Y' class fare which is two to four times the price of the cheapest economy ticket. In addition, you have to stay in a hotel of their choice for seven nights. If you get a hotel confirmation at all, it will be for a $40 to $50 room, for which you will be charged $125 a night for seven nights. And you must deal with a travel agency out-of-state by mail only, giving them at least 45 days notice of when you want to travel and three potential travel dates. Whatever dates you pick will likely not be available."

Guard Your Health

Be careful of your health in countries without modern sanitation. Call your county health department or discuss the destination with your travel agent. If there have been recent outbreaks of highly infectious diseases, they will be aware of that; you should procure innoculations if recommended. Do not drink the water in underdeveloped countries. Nor should you eat salads or fruit you cannot peel unless the hotel is a three-star or better and states that it has only purified water.

Political Upheavals

Our world is constantly changing. Countries undergo major political upheavals. Each month the U.S. State Department issues monthly travel advisory sheets. Your travel agent has them. Ask to see those sheets or ask your travel agent to study them for you. You will then be prepared. Travel advisory sheets also note information on the outbreak of certain diseases such as cholera, almost as soon as it happens, in any area of the world. Your ounce of prevention can then make your journey a healthy one.

Travel Light!

An old Spanish proverb states, "On a long journey even a straw weighs heavy." The less you travel with, the more unencumbered you will feel. It is not really necessary to take that hair dryer and the traveling iron. If you are traveling out of the United States or Canada, chances are the voltage will be different. Once I plugged in one of my American toys, a curling rod for my hair, using an adapter for the Austrian voltage. The entire floor of the small quaint hotel was instantly plunged into darkness which lasted for a couple of hours. I felt terrific guilt and now carry bobby pins.

You don't need to go out and buy a new wardrobe before you take a trip. Who will know that the dress or suit you are wearing at that elegant welcoming dinner at the beginning of the trip was purchased for your niece's wedding two years ago?

My sister recently returned from a trip to Russia. One man in her group wore a different outfit each day. Some of his concoctions were a bit outlandish, but he had raided Goodwill and St. Vincent de Paul secondhand stores before leaving the states. Each day he left his entire outfit behind in his hotel room as a generous tip to his maid, who doubtlessly found a relative who could wear the clothes. As his suitcases emptied, he purchased small gifts to take home and tucked them into his bag.

If you buy all new clothes you'll be very disappointed if the bag vanishes. Many a suitcase has ended up at the wrong destination. The majority are found in Paris when they should be in Munich and are eventually reunited with their owner. Help the airlines out by having a baggage tag with your name, home address and phone number clearly printed on it, in addition to the tag with your printed destination.

Inside your bag tape the same information, in case the baggage tag gets ripped off by a hungry goat waiting for his master in the airport. Leave a copy of your itinerary inside as well. If you are going to Athens before returning home, it would be far better if that suitcase caught up with you in Greece, rather than Des Moines. It might even be wise to leave a photostat copy of your passport and your airline ticket at home with a relative or friend.

Record Your Documents

Copy down the numbers of your airline ticket and your passport number as well and store these in some place safe in your luggage, along with the numbers of your traveler's checks. Such precautions can facilitate the issuing of new documents and aid you in recovering the money represented by those traveler's checks.

How Important is Fitness?

Do not feel you have to stop traveling if you can no longer walk the vast distances in the modern airports. I have been escorting groups to faraway areas of the world for ten years now. There are often two of my people who cannot manage the airport without wheelchair assistance. They have journeyed with me to Australia, New Zealand, many parts of Western Europe, to South America and to Kenya, as well as many places closer to California.

They are still able to walk, but not with flight bags and heavy coats the length of a modern airport. Airlines are accustomed to the request for wheelchair assistance for the elderly, or for those suffering from a painful hip problem or who are fighting arthritis. All over the world, courteous people meet the flights with the wheelchair and whisk one through customs, up elevators and through airport mazes to join the rest of the group of travelers.

If you can walk the length of a city block slowly, you can probably enjoy more than three-fourths of the soft adventures mentioned in this book. Two of the people with me on the Kenya safari were met in Amsterdam and Nairobi with wheelchairs at the end of long flights, but their thrill with the tour as they gazed out at the wild creatures gamboling about made my own pleasure more intense.

The Key: Flexibility

The key to successful travel is the same as for any of life's adventures. Flexibility is important. One must be able to bend like the bamboo in order to survive in today's rapidly changing world. Your schedule for meals and for all of your routines will be altered while you are traveling. Carry healthy snacks with you if you have to eat frequently for health reasons. Special dietary needs can be served on airlines and on cruises. Let your travel agent know these needs in advance.

Maintain a healthy open mind. Not every society's rules are the same as our own. The Zulus, for example, revere their elders, but must remain seated when an elder enters their area, so that they are lower than he is. They must push him aside and leave the hut first so as to protect him from an unknown enemy if he wishes to leave. Our training has taught us the exact opposite in both instances.

The Masai in Kenya are fascinating to watch and one longs to photograph them in their long colorful robes, but they are superstitious. They might chase your vehicle and throw a spear at you if you frighten them by taking their photo. We must respect their wishes.

A set of preconceived expectations and prejudices can weigh more heavily upon one than those electrical appliances. Travel with an open mind and you will experience the delight a small child has upon making a new discovery.

Enjoy people and places very unlike your own! Widen your horizons with travel. The world beyond our own backyard can bring a touch of wonder and magic into our lives.

Experience it fully. Try a new adventure next year. Reach within yourself, stretch and grow as you explore new horizons and find yourself exploring the inner space of the sea while snorkeling or scuba diving, or the clouds in space as you are floating away from earth for a brief hour in a hot air balloon.

The world is yours to enjoy, but not to despoil, to experience with joy, not fear, with trust and love, not distrust and hate. To travel is to broaden one's own horizons, to let in the light of understanding for various peoples and their cultures and to take pleasure in our very complex world. Take time out to discover that world beyond your own front porch.

Experience it through personal adventures rather than from the back seat of a crowded tour bus. Dare to live your life fully and enjoy it all!

Bon voyage!

ADDITIONAL TOUR OPERATORS
AND TRAVEL VENDORS

Write or call for information. Your travel agent may also have brochures from these companies.

AUSTRALIA-NEW ZEALAND

AAT King's Australian Adventure Tours
5693 Whitnall Highway
North Nollywood, CA 91601

Jetset Tours
1960 E. Grand Ave.#800
El Segundo, CA 90245

Tahiti Nui's Island Dreams
1750 Bridgeway #101-B
Sausalito, CA 94965   FAX (415)331-8309

Ted Cook/Islands in the Sun
760 W 16th St.#L
Costa Mesa, CA 92627   FAX (714)548-1654

CANADA-ALASKA

Alaska Discovery (wilderness adventures)
369-R So. Franklin St.
Juneau, AK 99801   (907)586-1911

Alaska Nature Tours
P.O. Box 491
Haines, AK 99827   (907)766-2876

Alaska Wildland Adventures (offers a Senior Safari)
P.O. Box 259
Trout Lake, WA 98650   (800)334-8730

Holland America/Westours
300 Elliott Ave.W.
Seattle, WA 98119   FAX (206)281-7110

DELUXE

Abercrombie and Kent Intl. Inc.
1420 Kensington Rd.
Oakbrook, IL 60521   FAX (708)954-3324

Society Expeditions Cruises   (see page 50)

EUROPE
Caravan Tours Inc.
    401 Michigan Ave.
    Chicago IL 60611   FAX (312)321-9810
Earth Ventures (bicycle tours in Europe/Australia)
    6608-B Saint James Dr.
    Indianapolis, IN 56217   (317)783-9449
Globus-Gateway/Cosmos
    150 S. Los Robles Ave.
    Pasadena, CA 91101   FAX (818)499-8856
Olson Travelworld
    100 N. Sepulveda Blvd.
    El Segundo, CA 90245
Slattery's Travel (gypsy caravan holidays in Ireland)
    1 Russell St.
    Tralee Co.
    Kerry, Ireland   066-26277
Ten-Speed Tours (bicycling through Europe)
    P.O. Box 7152
    Van Nuys, CA 91409   (818)786-4279
TWA-Getaway Vacations
    28 S Sixth St.
    Philadelphia, PA 19106   (800)438-2929

HAWAII
Classic Hawaii
    One N First St.
    San Jose, CA 95223   FAX (408)287-9272
Eye of the Whale (marine/wilderness adventures)
    P.O. Box 1269
    Kapa'au, HI 96755   (800)889-0227
Happi Tours Hawaii
    18800 Cox Ave.
    Saratoga, CA 95070   FAX (408)379-6751

Hawaii World
    2056 First St.
    Livermore, CA 94550   FAX (415)433-3677
Sunmakers
    P.O. Box 96045
    Bellevue, WA 98009   (800)841-4321

ORIENT

Innerasia Expeditions
    2627-T Lombard St.
    San Francisco, CA 94123   (800)551-1769
Pacific Delight
    132 Madison Ave.
    New York, NY 10016   (212)532-3406
Society Expeditions Cruises   (see page 503)

SOUTH AMERICA

Magellan Tours
    925 116th Ave. NE #215
    Bellevue WA 98004
Unique Adventures
    690 Market St. #1100
    San Francisco, CA 94104   FAX (415)986-1749

UNITED STATES

Cameras, Horses and Trails
    P.O. Box 219
    Powell, WY 82435   (307)645-3173
Close-up Expeditions (photographic adventures)
    c/o Lyon Travel Services
    1031 Ardmore Ave.
    Oakland, CA 94610   (415)465-8955
Elderhostel (also worldwide)
    75 Federal St.
    Boston, MA 02110

INDEX